"Anybody who is thinking of having any procedure should read *The Gift You Give Yourself*. Besides being a facial plastic surgeon, I have been a patient, and some of these thoughts have come across my mind, but . . . these incredible words . . . opened up another way of thinking of vitality, youth, and feeling great! . . . A must-read!"

—PAUL NASSIF, MD, FPS
Host of the Television Show *Botched*

"Demand for surgical and nonsurgical facial rejuvenation continues to grow, and social media is replete with self-serving claims and information lacking validity. *The Gift You Give Yourself*—authored by an insightful and seasoned practitioner of the art and science of facial surgery—is a welcome and refreshing change in that it provides the kind of information that serves to promote patient safety and inform prospective patients.

"Raising a scalpel to alter facial appearance is an awesome responsibility never to be taken lightly. Dr. McCollough makes this clear and goes on to describe the many benefits of the various procedures. Drawing on his extensive experience, and through patient testimonials, [he] illustrates that, beyond physical enhancement, facial surgery has the power to enrich and alter lives.

"This well-written, comprehensive, and easy-to-read book is not only a description of available options or a patient's guide; benefits [to facial surgery] beyond the physical changes are discussed in detail.

"Though the primary audience for this book is the general public, I feel all who undertake surgical enhancement will benefit from reading this book, especially those just embarking on their career."

—FOAD NAHAI, MD
Editor, *Aesthetic Surgery Journal*

"As a television executive, I learned the importance of a pleasing appearance in helping anchors and correspondents forge a bond with viewers. Dr. McCollough shows in *The Gift You Give Yourself* how important it is for everyone, not just those in the public eye, to gain the confidence that comes from feeling you are at your best. In down-to-earth language and with common-sense guidance, Dr. McCollough demonstrates that the body is inextricably linked to the mind and the spirit, that appearance is intertwined with health, and that caring for your body is the gift that will also nourish your feelings of self-worth."

—BARBARA COCHRAN
Curtis B. Hurley Chair of Public Affairs Journalism, Missouri School of Journalism
President Emeritus of RTNDA and RTNDF
Former Vice President of News, NPR

"After more than four decades of clinical practice and experience, Dr. McCollough connects all the dots of a comprehensive life plan for appearance enhancement.

"Dr. McCollough's lifework proves to be a tried and true recipe for well-being based on his own integrative model of mind, body, and spirit; self-assessment; and professional team consultation.

"*The Gift You Give Yourself* always keeps the focus on balance and moderation. Readers will celebrate Dr. McCollough's extraordinary awareness and insight!"

—SUSAN B. WILKIE MCHALE, PhD

"When my employees and patients participate in the recommendations offered in this book, they demonstrate a new confidence, increased energy, and enjoy looking as young as they feel."

—LARRY D. SHOEMAKER, MD, MBA, FAAFP
Former CEO of St. Joseph Hospital and Children's Hospital
CMO of Marshfield Clinic Health System, Marshfield, WI

"An erudite and inspirational game changer, allowing us to optimize our health through mind, body, and spirit . . . An absolute pathfinder ahead of its time."

—FIONA STEFFEN, CERTIFIED HEALER
UK National Federation of Spiritual Healers

"A sine qua non for charting one's course to personal appearance and health."

—HUGH JACKS
Proprietor, Potential Enterprises
Former President and CEO, BellSouth Services

THE GIFT
YOU GIVE
YOURSELF

THE GIFT
YOU GIVE
YOURSELF

Surgical and Other Choices That Enhance Your Appearance, Confidence, and Health

E. GAYLON McCOLLOUGH, MD, FACS

BROWN BOOKS
PUBLISHING GROUP

The Gift You Give Yourself
Surgical and Other Choices That Enhance Your Appearance, Confidence, and Health

Brown Books Publishing Group
Dallas, TX / New York, NY
www.BrownBooks.com
(972) 381-0009

A New Era in Publishing®

Publisher's Cataloging-In-Publication Data
Names: McCollough, E. Gaylon, author.
Title: The gift you give yourself : surgical and other choices that enhance your appearance, confidence, and health / E. Gaylon McCollough, MD, FACS.
Description: Dallas, TX ; New York, NY : Brown Books Publishing Group, [2020]
Identifiers: ISBN 9781612544342
Subjects: LCSH: Self-care, Health. | Surgery, Plastic. | Beauty, Personal. | Skin--Care and hygiene. | Nutrition.
Classification: LCC RA776.95 .M33 2020 | DDC 613--dc23

ISBN 978-1-61254-434-2
LCCN 2019915838

Printed in United States
10 9 8 7 6 5 4 3 2 1

For more information or to contact the author, please go to
www.McCulloughPlasticSurgery.com.

This book is dedicated to the tens of thousands of patients who trusted me with their appearance, health, and well-being.

You have within you, the resources to become the
shining example of humanity you were created to be.

—E. Gaylon McCollough, MD, FACS

Contents

Note From the Author — xv

Foreword — xvii

1: Becoming the Person of Your Dreams — 1

2: The Appearance Factor — 5

3: Your Personal Dream Team — 15

4: The Economics of Attractiveness — 23

5: How Old Are You? — 31

6: Beyond the Surface — 33

7: Nonsurgical Skin-Enhancement Products:
Help or Hype? — 39

8: The Weight Factor — 47

9: Smart Nutrition: Feeding Your Body — 61

10: The Effects of Hormones and Stress on Aging — 67

11: Enhancement Medicine and Surgery — 73

12: Nose-Enhancing Surgery:
The Rhinoplasty Operation — 81

13: Chin Enhancement — 87

14: Lip Enhancement: Lifting and Augmentation — 93

15: Corrective Surgery for Protruding Ears   99

16: Appearance-Enhancing Surgery:
     A Condition-Specific Perspective   103

17: A More Youthful Face:
     Before You Consent to Altering It   115

18: Sagging and Aging Eyelids:
     The Corrective Procedure Known as Blepharoplasty   129

19: Lifting the Aging and Drooping Eyebrow:
     The Pros and Cons   137

20: The Facelift Operation   141

21: The Rejuvenation Process:
     What You Might Not Otherwise Be Told   151

22: The Rest of the Skin-Rejuvenation Story   155

23: Chemical Peeling:
     A Time-Tested Elixir for Aging Skin   163

24: Dermabrasion: Another Skin-Resurfacing Technique   167

25: Laser-Assisted Skin Rejuvenation   171

26: Why Caring for Your Skin Helps Take Care of You   177

27: Treating Skin Cancer   189

28: Scar Revision and Skin Surgery   201

29: Surgical Body Contouring   209

30: Beyond the Breasts   217

31: The Male Factor   225

32: The Hair Factor   233

33: The Lifelong Value of Appearance Enhancement
    in Your Younger Years   249

34: Additional Self-Enhancement Measures   259

35: Feeling as Well as You Look:
    The Superior Doctor's Role   265

36: Your Body, in Shape, in All the Ways Possible   273

37: Your Enhancement Prescription   283

38: The Right and Wrong Reasons to Consult
    Appearance-Enhancing Professionals   293

39: Gifts for the Taking   301

    Acknowledgments   307

    Suggested Reading   309

    About the Author   310

NOTE FROM THE AUTHOR

My friend and best-selling author Andy Andrews makes a good point when he says that less than 5 percent of readers read the preface or foreword of books.[1]

I'd like to suggest that you follow the 5 percent's lead and read Dr. Jan Seward's foreword on the next page. Containing both professional and personal elements, her testimonial sets the stage for creating your own life-enhancement plan that—if consistently and vigilantly followed—could command the doors of opportunity to swing open for you, just as they have for thousands of patients I've had the honor of guiding toward becoming the person of their dreams.

---

1. Andy Andrews, *The Bottom of the Pool* (Nashville: W Publishing Group, 2019).

FOREWORD

The Gift You Give Yourself is beautifully written, thoroughly researched, and deeply inspiring.

I had the great good fortune of meeting Dr. McCollough twenty years ago as his patient. At that time, I was a psychologist in the field of natural and integrative medicine, and although I was aware of the powerful mind/body connection, I had never seen this knowledge so thoroughly integrated into the care and treatment of patients as I did with Dr. McCollough. Under his caring and capable hands, I experienced not just a cosmetically altering procedure but a life-altering experience.

Forty-six years into his career, Dr. McCollough continues to inspire, shape, and change lives from the inside out. He is a true exemplar of the adage that beauty is so much more than skin deep. How we feel on the inside is always reflected on the outside, and the world responds to our feelings as surely as to the looks on our faces. By addressing the whole person—body, mind, and spirit—Dr. McCollough makes his patients whole.

The Gift You Give Yourself is a treasure—the collection of a life's work of study and practice now generously shared with the world. Students of aesthetic medicine and surgery can use it for a handbook. Experienced practitioners in the field should as well. Patients—former or current—will find, as I did, that their experience of healing will improve upon reading and absorbing the all-important lessons of this book: our thoughts create our lives, and changing our thoughts for the better changes our lives for the better in every way. It's that simple—and that profound.

Dr. Jan Seward, PsyD, MCAT
Clinical Instructor of Psychology and Integrative Health,
University of Bridgeport College of Naturopathic Medicine;
Life Management Practitioner, Department of Health and Healing,
Canyon Ranch Resorts and Spa,
Lenox, Massachusetts

CHAPTER 1

Becoming the Person of Your Dreams

Have you ever dreamed of becoming a more appealing, healthier, and more confident version of yourself? How much do you want to see that dream come true? What measures are you willing to take to make it happen? Are you open to considering the same prescriptive advice and methods that I have recommended to thousands of patients—and continue to do so in my practice on a daily basis? If your answer is yes, you have taken the first step toward giving yourself the gifts that thousands of my patients have given to themselves: a more appealing appearance and the multiple benefits that accompany it.

Did you know that when you look your best, you are also more likely to experience an improvement in your health? Would you like to see the doors of opportunity open more frequently and wider than before—doors that lead to interpersonal relationships, career advancement, and more?

As an improved version of you begins to take shape, you will see how making powerful—and lasting—first impressions instantly places you ahead of the competition, whoever they might be and whatever the arena in which you're competing. This is not a new reality. In fact, Aristotle was the first to record that "a pleasing appearance is more important than any letter of introduction." This celebrated Greek philosopher provided a lesson that has proven to span the ages: the way you look when you meet someone is more important than any document or diploma you bring with you, even if the recommendation is written on your behalf by a prominent or famous advocate.

To underscore Aristotle's lesson on first impressions, let me share a scenario involving Michelangelo, another iconic artisan. As the story goes, Michelangelo was in the process of bargaining with a stone merchant for a large piece of marble. Once the intense negotiations were settled, a fascinated bystander approached Michelangelo and asked, "Why are you willing to pay so much for an oversized rock?"

To which the artist replied, "Can't you see it? There is an angel confined inside that piece of marble, and I must set it free."

Michelangelo's lesson rivals the one that Aristotle penned. Both of them reinforce the central theme of this book. In more ways than we might imagine, you and I are sculptors. Our minds, bodies, and spirits are divinely given to us so that we can enhance them. We have it within us to cast off our self-imposed restrictions as well as the constraints imposed upon us by society. If you choose to faithfully and diligently exercise that gift, the person inside you that was always waiting to be freed will emerge from within these limitations.

Becoming the person of your dreams is a process—one that is on-going and fraught with challenges and distractions both expected and unexpected. You would be wise to assemble a team of professionals to assist you. This book explains how. For as long as you continue reading, I offer to serve as your adviser, coach, and cheerleader.

As a physician and surgeon who honors the Hippocratic oath, I feel obliged to share with you the truths that have been revealed to me on the way to becoming a metaphysician and surgeon. I will also address the skillfully packaged hype about appearance enhancement being propagated to an unsuspecting public by a masterfully created and massively funded marketing campaign. Sadly, that campaign extends into the once-revered halls of medicine, mainstream media, and institutions of higher learning.

Throughout my career, I have paid close attention as scores of so-called "miracle" cures came and went from the landscape of my industry. Without equivocation, I can say that many more "too good to be true" discoveries fall by the wayside of false promise than endure the tests of time. Like previous generations of consumers, you are being fed an ever-mounting mass of misinformation, anecdotal results, and inflated promises. In my experience, many of the alternatives presented to consumers by a large segment of the appearance and health enhancement industrial complex serve the industry (or the designated reporting outlet) more than they serve the consumer.

The fact that you were drawn to this book means that you might be a potential consumer of products, services, and procedures that claim to enhance your appearance and thus your well-being. It could also mean that you are a fact finder, dedicated to discovering the truth and sharing it with your audience. Either scenario means that you are entitled to a truthful and comprehensive perspective on the products, procedures, and machines that too often provide more hype than hope.

Some of my fellow appearance-enhancing colleagues will likely view this book as a challenge to their efforts. Companies that manufacture or sell overly hyped devices and machines will agree with them. From start to finish, I have made it my mission to see that the revelations I share and the concerns I raise are intended for the enlightenment of patients and clients, who place their faces, bodies, and lives in the hands of those of us they have been learned to trust.

So if you are open to becoming a better-informed consumer or provider of appearance- and health-enhancing services and products . . . if you are willing to demand more of your appearance and health enhancement professionals and products than you might have previously imagined . . . if you are prepared to learn things about the industry that have been stealthily kept from you, let's pull back the curtain and shine the light of truth on all the hype. In the process, let's also embark on an honest analysis of the "you" that you currently believe you are—inside and out. Let's explore the boundless gifts you have been given so that you can give an enhanced version of each talent right back to yourself, particularly the talents that will allow you to set yourself free from any and all previous versions of the person you are today.

You are currently a newly created version of the person you were years ago. Each cell in your body is a closely related clone of the cell it replaced. How closely it mirrors its parent cell depends on the thoughts you harbor in your mind and the lifestyle choices you make. New cells are not necessarily perfect clones. They can be exact replicas, enhanced replicas, or less healthy replicas. As I explain in the pages to follow, it's up to you which of these three alternatives comprise the new you. The next chapter explains how to become the master of the cell-replication process taking place within your body and how to create the mind-set and lifestyle that will convert healthy and beautiful thoughts into a beautifully balanced body, mind, spirit, and life. The sculptor in you will reveal to the world the version of yourself that you choose to be.

Dr. Orison Swett Marden once referred to doctors who seek solutions beyond traditional methods as metaphysicians. Nearly a century after Dr. Marden coined the term, Catherine Collautt, PhD, professor of European Union and employment law at the University of Cambridge, defined a metaphysician as "a practicing healer/adviser that changes physical reality by working with the principles and powers and 'things' that underlie it, and especially the mind or psyche." It is from that same perspective that I publish the observations and recommendations you'll find throughout this book. As a metaphysician and surgeon, I view it as my responsibility to monitor the new products and procedures that come to the market-places of appearance and health. If they prove to be effective, I include them in the services I offer to my patients.

As a pragmatist, I will not profess to have all the answers. To the contrary, I am constantly looking for better ways to help my patients realize their dreams. My intent is to provide to you, the reader, the same kind of advice that I give to each patient who consults with me on a firsthand basis. Like them, you'll also be asked to consider the same admonitions. This is all for the purpose of helping you give yourself the gift that is yours for the making—a life lived well for more years than would have otherwise been yours to enjoy.

With those thoughts in mind, let's get started.

CHAPTER 2

The Appearance Factor

I begin this chapter with an actual encounter that I had with a patient who consulted me for appearance-enhancing surgery.

"Before meeting with you, I reviewed the photographs my assistant took this morning," I said to the woman sitting on the opposite side of the desk in my consultation room. "I have some thoughts I will share with you when we go over to the three-way mirror on the wall. However, before we do so, I'd like for you to answer a few questions."

The prospective patient nodded in agreement.

"To give you a heads-up, I'm going to ask them all at once. Then we'll go back and revisit each question individually."

Again, she nodded and said, "I understand." My questions to her were:

- What do you hope to achieve by undergoing appearance-enhancing surgery?
- When did you decide it was time to enhance your appearance?
- Did someone say something to you that tipped the scales?
- If so, what relationship do you have with that person?
- Who will be happiest with a younger, healthier, better-looking version of you?
- If we come to terms with the procedures that I believe will help you achieve your goals, are you prepared to follow my advice before and after the procedures we agree upon, including professionally administered skin and health care?

My prospective patient appeared a bit taken aback by my line of questioning and responded with a question of her own.

"May I ask how much psychology training you have had?"

I smiled and thought to myself, *One of my facial plastic surgery mentors called what we do "psychological surgery." As such, we are bound to treat the minds of our patients as much as we treat their faces, necks, eyelids, and noses.*

Now imagine that the person sitting on the opposite side of my consultation desk is *you*. How would you answer the questions I posed? Be honest with yourself, because becoming a better-looking, healthier, and happier you is not a quick fix. Nor is it a permanent solution. Rather, maintaining an appealing appearance is an ongoing *process* that likely includes both surgical and nonsurgical solutions. In that regard, looking your best on an ongoing basis requires a partnership of like-minded professionals. It also calls for commitment (and cooperation) from all parties involved: your surgeon, your personal physician, your skin-care expert, your hair stylist, your wardrobe consultant, your family, your closest friends, and—most of all—*you*, the central focus of your dreams.

Perhaps you are one of the fortunate few to whom a perfect appearance was awarded from the outset. You were born beautiful. You were a beautiful baby and a prom queen or king. You were Miss This or Mr. That—but time and not-so-wise personal decisions have changed all that once was yours. If you are to remain beautiful or handsome, you must be willing to accept the facts of life and do the things that are required to keep you so. But perhaps you are like the majority of us. Mother Nature did not bless you with a perfectly shaped face, nose, or body. If that is the case, you have the potential within you to do something about that too.

In both cases, becoming the best you possible is a matter of exercising the one gift that you, I, and our fellow human beings were all given: the gift that allows us to recognize the talents and assets we were given and the resources at our disposal in order to choose those that fit our own talents and objectives and to then—with the assistance of trained professionals—turn the potential we were given at birth into a reality of our own making.

This is the miracle of *free will*. If you choose to follow the recommendations I set forth in this book, you will be able to prove to yourself and to the world around you that you are not only capable of mastering your thoughts but committed to being the best you possible, physically, mentally, and spiritually. You are committed to becoming the person of your dreams in all measurable ways. When you make such a commitment, the ripple (or butterfly) effect comes into play. Your decision will impact others and encourage them to follow your lead. Imagine such a world—a world in which everyone puts their best face and body forward every day; a world in which every human being becomes the best that they are capable of becoming. Above all, imagine that you have it within you to help create such a world. Imagine that there are professionals who can help you do these things.

* * *

Now, I'd like for you to answer the questions I posed to the prospective patient referenced at the beginning of this chapter.

- What do you hope to achieve by undergoing appearance-enhancing procedures?
- When did you decide it was time to enhance your appearance?
- Did someone say something to you that tipped the scales?
- If so, what relationship do you have with that person?
- Who will be happiest with a younger, healthier, better-looking version of you?
- If we come to terms with the procedures I or the surgeon you choose believes will best achieve your goals, are you willing to follow your surgeon's advice before and after the procedures agreed upon, including professionally managed skin and health care?

In preparation for learning about the procedures, products, and mechanical devices designed to improve your appearance and health, I ask that you thoughtfully answer the questions posed above.

Human beings like you represent achievers—an ever-growing number of people who possess the grit to convert their wildest dreams into reality. The fact that you are still reading indicates that you identify with those of us who are also dreamers and enablers of dreams that come true.

I offer the advice and counsel of this book in order to assist you in your journey and address false—or exaggerated—claims about the benefits of applying a certain commercially available product to your skin, swallowing a combination of pills and capsules, following a certain commercialized diet, or becoming a participant in some scheme that might have been implanted in your mind by profit-driven companies and professionals.

Becoming aware of these facts and then adopting and adhering to the mind-set that you are a participant in ensuring your health and well-being is a gift that you can give yourself. It is the first—and, I contend, the most crucial—step toward achieving dreams that you might have never before imagined.

The evening after I met with the woman mentioned at the beginning of this chapter, I reflected on conversations with other patients I had seen—and cared for—earlier that day.

- One was a recent widower in his early seventies who was just a few days from a face and neck lift.
- Another was an unmarried professional woman (an accountant in her late fifties) who was a few days out from a maintenance face and eyelid tuck that included a skin-resurfacing procedure to address the newly acquired wrinkles in her facial skin.
- Then there was a teenage girl whose nose I had corrected a few months back. During the visit that day, she told me not only that she was pleased with the appearance of her new nose but that the breathing difficulties and frequent headaches from which she suffered were no longer a problem.
- There was the wife of a dentist who—according to her—had long wanted to have rejuvenating facial surgery but had been too apprehensive to take the first step, at least not until her husband suggested that she schedule a consultation with me.
- There was the CEO of a national company who had undergone facial and eyelid plastic surgery several months before. That day, she had sent over a set of postoperative photographs for my review and comments.
- Then there was the prospective patient who slipped by my four-plus decades of experience in screening realistically driven candidates

for appearance-enhancing surgery. This was a patient who would never be satisfied with the changes made to her face and body, no matter how they were performed; a patient who would ultimately manifest all the signs and symptoms of body dysmorphic disorder (BDD), a condition I address in chapter 38.

As I struggled to shut down my racing mind, I thought, "There are things missing from today's interactions with my patients . . ."

I had not received a call from the assistant of the queen of one of the Middle Eastern nations asking me to cancel appointments with established patients and fly up to Atlanta to conduct a secret consultation with her queen.

I had not received a call from one of America's top country and pop entertainers who'd insisted that I break my rules on preoperative laboratory testing and medical clearance from his personal physician.

I had not received a request from a doctor who had served a postgraduate fellowship in facial plastic surgery with me and who had asked me to, in essence, falsify a form he needed to obtain a license in another state.

I had not acted upon an urge to challenge a television network that had aired documercials earlier that day promoting too-good-to-be-true products and procedures by responding, "Whatever happened to evidence-based science? When—if ever—will truth in advertising become the standard when referencing mind-, body-, and spirit-enhancing products and procedures?"

I had received an emailed photograph of a patient and friend upon whom I had repaired a skin cancer defect a few weeks previously. Over the past couple of days, she had noticed a bit of irritation of the skin in the regions and wanted to know what to do.

I had received an eConsult request from a woman who had suffered with cystic acne as a teenager and been left with unsightly scars on the lower third of her face. She had undergone laser therapy on the scars performed by a colleague who either did not know that laser therapy would not make any appreciable improvement on her scars or took advantage of the patient's naivety.

Perhaps these reflections can help you gain a broader perspective of the appearance- and health-enhancement industry and the challenges we face. With these insights in mind, you can now proceed through the pages that follow with insight into what it means to be an appearance- and health-enhancing metaphysician and why I am compelled to share the things I have learned over the past half century with you. My only request is that you pay forward what you learn and share it with those you care for and about.

**

In keeping with the underlying theme of this book, it occurred to me that when any body owner hands off the divinely endowed gift that was given to them at the time of their birth, the body owner's destiny no longer lies in their own hands. They are no longer the master of their own self. I once read a line from a book of quotations that makes this point. Though I paraphrase, the resonating message is the same: "When *you* are in charge of a journey, you can embark upon it—or change course—when *you* choose. When others are involved, you will leave—or change courses—when *others* choose." This truism also applies to your own journey of lifestyle management.

In keeping with the practice of reaching back into my memory bank of thoughts, ideas, admonitions, and platitudes, I offer another axiom: everything happens for a reason. No truer words were ever spoken. The metascientist Sir Isaac Newton is credited with the theory of cause and effect, meaning that for every effect, there is an underlying cause. I trust that you, the reader, will come away from what you are about to read with the following conclusion: the "reason" for what happened to you is, more often than not, based upon thoughts that you, as a body owner, allowed to set up shop within your mind. Harbored thoughts become self-fulfilling prophecies. Good thoughts—positive thoughts—tend to cause good things to happen to the mind, body, and spirit. On the other hand, negative thoughts tend to lead to disappointment, ill health, and failure. A related truism to consider is, "Whether you think you *can* or *cannot*, you are right almost every time."

If you accept the gift I referred to in previous paragraphs—the one you were given to give right back to yourself—and develop it to its maximum potential, your efforts will assist you in clearing obstacles, embarking on the journey to become the person of your dreams when the time is right for you, and traveling the course that proves itself to be the best route to the desired end result. This gift is known by many descriptive terms. For the purpose of this treatise, I choose to refer to it as *self-mastery*: the ability to direct our bodies, minds, and spirits toward becoming everything that each component of our being is capable of becoming. That talent[2] (gift) was awarded to the human species by our Creator(s), the "us" and "our" referenced in Genesis 1:26: "And God said, Let us make man in our image, after our likeness" (King James Version).

Based upon decades of research and thoughtful logic, I contend that every person is an "us" and an "our," as we are all created by a team of heavenly based Creators—"in the beginning" and since—with God as the captain and coach.

With any talent awarded to us (individually and collectively) also comes a commitment to maintaining each component of what makes us "human" (mind, body, and spirit) in good working order for as long as possible. As this relates to handing off the reasons why things happen to anyone other than oneself, I offer the following.

Maybe you are a body owner who, early in your life, set out to become the best you could be in a particular field with an idea that jumped into your head during a moment of inspiration. In those developmental days, you realized that to achieve your personal best, you would need assistance from those who already knew the answers to the questions reverberating in your mind. First you started to consult your family,

2. See the Parable of the Talents, Matthew 25:14–30.

friends, coaches, and spiritual advisers. As you began to experience success and your aspirations became greater in scope, you expanded your circle of advisers. Some of them you could meet with on a personal basis. Others you could only consult by pouring through the annals of history. As you received positive feedback, you built up enough confidence to grow and evolve organically, or maybe you were lucky enough to land a patron mentor who coaxed you up the ladder of fulfillment for a while. You reached out to anyone you thought might be able to help you become the person you came to realize you were always meant to be. But now the time for short-term solutions is over. You came to realize that the gift you were given by the Source of your creation at the time of your conception is greater than you might have originally imagined, but you also realized that to take advantage of that gift and become your personal best, you would need professional guidance. Or perhaps you are among a rare group of human beings who have done all the right things to enhance their minds, bodies, and spirits. You've achieved things beyond your wildest imagination. You are locally, regionally, nationally, and internationally known as one of the best in your chosen field. Or perhaps . . .

- You are already one of the most beautiful or handsome individuals on the planet.
- You are already one of the best athletes in your chosen sport; but each morning, when you look into your bathroom mirror, you ask yourself, "Can I be—am I expected to be—even better?"
- You see a face and body that are beginning to exhibit the signs of aging.
- Your hair is thinning or turning gray.
- Your face is becoming etched with wrinkles.
- You are seeing loose skin and bags around your eyes, along your jawline, or in your neck.
- Your abdomen is no longer flat and "ripped."
- You legs and arms are beginning to show early signs of cellulite (clumping fat cells with spaces in between).

- If you are a woman, perhaps your breasts are sagging. If you are a man, perhaps you are seeing development of female-like breasts as a result of lower testosterone levels.
- You do not feel as energetic or fulfilled as you once did when you gaze into the mirror.
- You are not bounding up and down stairs as you once could.

Each of these observations indicates that the ever-advancing clock of time is taking its toll on your body and mind . . . and perhaps on your spirit, the third component of the triad of human experience. But if you are going to realize your dreams, what measures must you take? The next chapter provides answers.

CHAPTER 3

Your Personal Dream Team

The answer to "What can you do to recapture your youth and give yourself the opportunity to fulfill your remaining dreams?" is not that complicated. Assemble a team of advisers and experts who are willing to buy into your own dreams and capable of producing gold-medal results in the game of life.

As your life-enhancement plans are being developed, you should share with your team a warts-and-all perspective of your past life choices and experiences. Reveal to them the talents you once enjoyed, and measure their responses and promises. Do not be bashful. Withholding vital thoughts and information is not to your advantage. You should also share with your team the lesser talents that you possess and the failures you experienced while stretching the limits of your abilities. In short, the professionals on your team need to know about your more youthful years—the successes and failures you experienced. As I often say to my own patients, I can't fix it if I don't know about it. In a similar manner, your dream team will do a better job of helping you reach your potential if they know about your past experiences.

If they are to help you fully develop the gifts you were given at the time of your birth and help you become the person of your dreams, they should have unlimited access to the facts that led you to become the person you currently are. They should know if . . .

- You were once the dominant player in your profession—the one to whom people of all ages looked for advice and counsel.
- You previously had a solid operational plan in place and a like-minded team that bought into your dream and knew how to help you achieve it.
- Your original team of appearance- and health-enhancement professionals was steadily opening doors and supporting your efforts. Perhaps now some of those team members are beginning to give

in to the distractions that come with the aging process, or perhaps circumstances in their lives are becoming a distraction. As a result, they are falling behind on their responsibilities or are out of touch with the new evidence-based research that could—and should—replace the procedures, products, and processes of their era.

Perhaps you . . .

- Are beyond the age of forty, better informed than in your youth about both the new developments and the tried, tested, and true methods being propagated by the appearance- and health-enhancement industry.
- Are beginning to recognize changes in your mirror, in photographs (such as the way your clothes fit), and in having the stamina to carry out activities that once came easily.
- Recognize that two distinctively different choices lie ahead. Either you can accept the end-of-life circumstances that every human faces and retire gracefully into the sunset of life, or you can choose to be a fighter, an overachiever, a proven winner in whatever arenas you once competed.

With those thoughts in mind, you will be in a better position to enhance the gifts that you were given. As one of your life coaches, I challenge you to make a commitment to yourself. For as long as you are physically and mentally capable, pledge to . . .

- Resurrect and embrace the youthful juices that once flowed through your body and energized your mind.
- Embark upon the next step toward self-care and finding your place in the universe—the place and circumstances you choose to create to your own liking and capabilities.

I will not tell you that becoming the person of your dreams will be easy. In fact, it will require a commitment to set aside some of your current, comfortable lifestyle choices—the ones that have led you to become the person that you currently are. As one of your life-enhancement coaches, I am obliged to bring into the process a definition of "insanity" once offered by Albert Einstein. History recognizes him as one of the most brilliant minds that ever inhabited a human body, not only because of his theory of relativity but because he defined "insanity" as "continuing to do the same thing and expect a different result."

As you now know, I am a fan of the adage "everything happens for a reason." I believe Albert Einstein happened for a reason. I believe you happened for a reason. Throughout this book, I connect the words "reason" and "happens." In that regard, I suggest that there is a reason you were drawn to this book. There is a reason that professional advice from a dream team of consultants and providers is now yours to either ignore or make use of. That you are still reading suggests that you are more inclined to make changes happen for all the right reasons. If they happen, it is because you chose, of your own free will, to make them happen.

Although at present you might bring a treasure trove of wisdom to the game of life, finding the right place for an enlightened, rejuvenated, and reinvigorated you to show the world what is possible will require a wiser way forward. You must stop doing the same insane things that led you to lag behind classmates, siblings, and coworkers who look younger, have more energy, and are still more productive than you are. Lagging behind them in life's marathon means that you have some catching up to do. You must invest the same amount of time, energy, and resources that you invested in your younger, more energetic, and highly productive years. The revised lifestyle to which you must commit requires that you choose to harbor only youthful and healthy thoughts and choose to engage only in productive actions.

If, during the prime of your life, you were identified as an achiever, leader, or champion, you had to have chosen to become a significant force in a world that favors success. Although years have passed, you should not delay in setting aside a lifestyle that was, perhaps, rooted in Einstein's definition of insanity. Choose a different way forward—one that will assist you in achieving dreams that are both reasonable and within reach. Some of you can achieve your dreams on your own; some of you will require the assistance of a dream team. The bottom line is this: make the wise decision. If you require help, seek help. Doing so is a sign of wisdom and strength, not a sign of weakness.

If, with becoming an enhanced version of yourself at the forefront of your mind, you feel you need assistance, you should make the appropriate appointments and present your new life plan to a carefully selected team of professionals who claim to be able to assist you in becoming all that you can be—for the remainder of your life. With members of your team, hands are shaken, and, where appropriate, covenant-like hugs are exchanged. You sign a term sheet giving part of your well-being over your new best friend and leader of your team of counselors and caregivers.

As a body, mind, and spirit consult to thousands of people just like you, the advice I offer is this: never relinquish full control of your dreams. You are your body's owner and caretaker. Therefore, *you—and you alone*—are responsible for contacting and contracting with like-minded *partners* who are willing and able to assist you in developing the gifts that you were given to their maximum potential. You should not be seeking the advice of professionals who might be more interested in furthering *their own dreams* over yours.

If you hand off full control and fail to select the right team of professionals to be part of your life-enhancement venture, the results that you thought would take forty-five days might drag into six-plus months. Your life-enhancement team of professional might keep finding issues that lead to less-than-promised results and the renegotiating of terms. The relationship with those to whom you have entrusted your life and well-being might start to turn adversarial, especially if you haven't experienced the results you were promised.

Perhaps your life-management team's attention is focused on adding an endless menagerie of products, procedures, and services to your life-enhancement plan. In the back of your mind, remember that the "enhancement industry" is big business—so all profit-driven caveats apply.

Perhaps the resources you had planned to commit to giving yourself the best body, face, and mind possible are beginning to wear thin. You're losing sleep, seeing your financial resources dwindling, and beginning to distrust the individuals in whom you placed your trust. If so, you must confront the problem and the problem makers. Chapters toward the end of this book provide advice on how and when to take such actions.

Coming to the realization that *your* dreams are taking second place to those of members of your current professional team, you make it clear that you are disappointed with the outcome of the advice you have paid for. Immediately, the leader of your life-enhancement team replaces some key members of the team. According to the failed team leader, this new team has a completely different focus from that of the previous team members. They want to streamline the plan and create new efficiencies. You are beginning to think that you are part of some research project and self-promotion on the part of the professionals who are supposed to be focused on enhancing *your* appearance, health, and well-being. The "team" doesn't seem to "get" the image of you that you had in mind or be willing to invest time and expertise in seeing your dream become reality.

At this point, you have a selection of choices: to walk away and forfeit your dreams; to relentlessly press the issue until you are linked with the absolute most qualified and ethical professionals within the network (to who you give your trust); or to seek advice elsewhere. In either case, *the trust factor* between the care providers and the recipient has been strained . . . and is in jeopardy of becoming irreconcilable. The lifelong caregiver-patient relationship initially dreamed of takes a nosedive.

Six months later, every professional on the life-enhancement team is referring you to a colleague who is "better trained" to handle your specific needs and desires. And, with the interruption of continuity, many of the gains made are lost. Once again, you are on your own. You do not give up; rather, you exercise the gift provided to every one of us at the time of our birth—free will, the ability to choose one's own destiny.

You . . .

- Return to the proverbial drawing board.
- Search for like-minded friends, professionals, and institutions.
- Visit the internet and conduct evidence-based research.
- Read self-help books.
- Foolishly try any product, procedure, or technology that appears to make sense.

Still, you feel alone in your quest to become the person of your dreams, the one that you were always intended to be. Ultimately, creative thinking comes to a standstill. And in desperation, you picked up this book. While reading it . . .

- You discovered that the answers to the vast majority of your questions were there all along—that to become the person you were always intended to be, you only needed to recognize the gift that you had been given, the same gift that you were given to turn around and give back to yourself.
- You come to realize that when you reach out to God (the Source) and pray, you are also calling forward the part of God instilled *in you* when, like the metaphorical Adam and Eve, you were created "in [his] image" (Gen. 1:26, KJV).

Although, as is the case with many journeys, this one might seem a bit complex, there is an unrecognized and unappreciated *reason* for the journey you and I have been exploring as well as for the one upon which we are about to embark. There is a reason you were drawn to this book; a reason I was compelled to write it; a reason our minds intersected on this planet at this time in history. Go ahead and accept this truth: that you are reading these words absolutely *happened for a reason*, and that reason will be forthcoming in the pages that follow.

When you begin to see the you of your dreams coming into view, I'd like to believe that you will better understand the immeasurable powers that you possess. You will recognize and accept your God-given ability to identify and develop the talents awarded to you at the moment of conception. Then you will pay forward those gifts by, through your actions, demonstrating to your fellow human beings the best way to convert right-minded thoughts into a life defined by health, happiness, prosperity, and longevity.

During the process, you and I will also explore a subject that confronts us as a species—the species created in God's image. Once a body owner comes of age, who—other than the body owner—is responsible for their welfare and well-being? I contend that we are expected to contemplate this question and then, with the guidance provided in the voluminous annals of history and self-help, accept the responsibility for our actions (or lack of actions) in realms beyond our current understanding.

Now that this divinely commissioned challenge—that is, the expectation to multiply the talents awarded to each of us to their maximum potential—has been defined, let's explore how you, I, and fellow human beings arising from a wide variety of backgrounds already possess the secrets to a master plan that allows us to create a life of our own choosing.

In the next chapter, we begin to connect the dots. I'll demonstrate how your appearance is positively affected by improving your health and how your health can be improved by doing the things required to enhance your appearance. It is a connection that has yet to be considered by the so-called mainstream health-care systems available to the human race today.

CHAPTER 4

The Economics of Attractiveness

A few years back, a woman in her early sixties sat across my consultation from me. After we discussed her overall health, I asked her the question that—in one way or the other—I pose to each of my patients, regardless of age, profession, or social status. "Can you share with me, in your own words, why you are here to see me?"

The woman replied with a common answer. "I'm really not sure. I am a recent widow and—because I am looking older than my fellow workers—in the next couple of years, I will be facing mandatory retirement from a job that I've held for most of my professional life. I have no interest in retiring and feel that if I am to be more competitive in a world that traditionally rewards youth and assumes that young people are more technologically savvy, I need to look younger than how I now look."

That woman's answer was the perfect segue for me to share with her (and you) what my four and a half decades of experience and evidence-based research have demonstrated. I responded to her revealing comments by sharing documented facts. Each year, the world over, millions of people undergo appearance-enhancing procedures. To their credit, each person seeking enhancement has concluded that improving their appearance is a time-tested way to make an investment *in themselves*. I shared with the woman seeking my counsel that she was not alone in her quest. Just like her, many men and women who had lost a spouse through death or divorce chose to undergo procedures of a cosmetic nature—cosmetic meaning that the procedures required to achieve the results she sought would be purely elective in nature and that, unfortunately, her existing health-care plan would not cover the associated costs. Thus, the financial responsibility of giving her a renewed sense of self-confidence would, unfortunately, fall outside her health-care plan.

Although it was not the response she wanted to hear, it was the truth—a truth that every colleague who offers appearance-enhancing procedures is obliged to share with his or her patients.

In keeping with the aforereferenced caveat I learned from my mentors, I informed the patient sitting before me that this category of professional services (cosmetic or appearance-enhancing surgery) is generally provided *outside* government-regulated health care, and these procedures are not covered by any health-insurance plans. In short, appearance-enhancing surgery, products, and procedures are gifts that women and men from all walks of life choose to give themselves—and when combined with the right mind-set, they generally deliver on the investment committed to the anticipated result.

Had the woman sitting before me been there following an accident, tumor surgery, or a congenital defect, I would have told her that the type of surgery she needed often qualified as "reconstructive" in nature and might qualify for coverage by government and private health-care plans. I emphasize the word *might* because the facts are these: increasingly, health plans are erroneously—and for self-serving reasons—calling clearly reconstructive procedures cosmetic in nature. By doing so, the company can deny—or greatly delay—the coverage their clients deserve.

Since they did not apply to her, I also chose not to address the current government and contract-specific regulations facing people of all ages, creeds, and races. However, as a potential candidate for insurance-related reconstructive surgery, you should have access to the big picture of health care as it exists today and will likely exist in the years to come. As a metaphysician and surgeon, I view it as my responsibility to make you aware of the changes coming to the health-care system as Americans know it.

The reason people of all ages and backgrounds choose to have purely elective appearance-enhancing surgery and pay for it without the assistance of their health-care insurance can be found in an often quoted study performed by *Psychology Today* in the early 1970s. The results of that research were made known to me by the late Dr. Jack Anderson, one of my highly respected mentors. According to Dr. Anderson's interpretation of the research, 40 percent of Americans were dissatisfied with the shape of their noses and 25 percent were dissatisfied with their chins (which, for many people, includes their neck). In my own practice, a third of all cosmetic procedures are performed on men. That percentage is steadily increasing.

It might surprise you to learn that the people (both male and female) who choose to undergo appearance-enhancement procedures are the same individuals who:

- Exhibit good posture and a quality I refer to as "countenance."
- Thoughtfully pay attention to their weight.
- Embrace healthy diets and take nutritional supplements only in the doses indicated by scientific testing.
- Engage in physical activity that tones and strengthens muscles and cardiovascular and pulmonary health.
- Maintain hormones (with professional assistance) at levels consistent with those of a youthful version of themselves.
- Visit a medical spa for relaxation and professional skin care.
- Augment their diets with pharmaceutical-grade vitamins and supplements.
- Whiten their teeth.
- Wear a smile on their face.
- Coordinate their clothes and accessories.
- Routinely groom their hair.
- Engage in personal and career-oriented activities that enhance the mind and spirit as well as the body.
- Associate with others—at work or at play—who have adopted similar lifestyle habits.

I suggest that you review the list of health- and appearance-enhancing lifestyle habits listed above. As you do so, you will quickly realize that none of them require cosmetic (aesthetic) surgery. Enhancing your appearance can begin with the proverbial flip of your thought processes. You can simply *choose* to adopt the lifestyle habits I suggest and watch the world look at you with a more favorable eye.

At some point, elective appearance-enhancing surgery might—or might not—enter the picture.

As you go about your daily activities, notice that attractive people appear to be happier people. You will also see that people who appear to be happy make you want to be in their presence. Regardless of age differences, attractive people are attracted *to other attractive people.*

Look around you, and you will see that love, luck, confidence, fame, and fortune tend to favor the person who presents a more pleasing appearance—and do not discount the "countenance factor." You will also notice that more attractive people tend to attract attractive people, enjoy life, have more energy, appear healthier, and exude the impression of confidence and power.

When making this point to my own patients, I use the example of the late actor Telly Savalas. When you apply Leonardo da Vinci's criteria for beauty or handsomeness to Telly's face, nothing fits, including the fact that the only hairline he had was the one that went from side to side just above his ears. However, Telly Savalas possessed an attribute that the faces of many Leonardo-perfect individuals lack. He displayed *countenance*, and because he did, he found himself in the presence of beautiful women.

You will see that while the majority of appearance-enhancing procedures are performed on women, *men* who might not measure up to the fame and countenance of Telly Savalas comprise the fastest-growing segment of people looking to improve the way they look.

Some would ask, "Why would an otherwise healthy individual elect to undergo elective surgery, knowing that the possibility of potentially serious problems exists?" The answer is this: it is a risk that generally pays *huge dividends* in interpersonal relationships and in the workplace. Said another way, appearance-enhancing procedures have the potential to improve the quality of a person's life beyond the nonsurgical alternatives addressed in previous paragraphs.

During consultation—and in my consumer-information book *The Appearance Factor*, which I provide to prospective patients—I use the example that when you embark upon a trip and fasten your seat belt in an automobile or airplane, you accept the reality that unthinkable things could happen to yourself and fellow passengers during the trip. However, because the odds of arriving safely at one's destination are monumentally greater than not, the vast majority of patients seeking appearance-enhancing surgery are more than willing to accept those risks—especially if the appearance-enhancing surgery they seek is performed by a reputable surgeon in a reputable facility.

Political correctness aside, today's America is a youth-oriented, competitive society with a strong emphasis on appearance. It is documented fact that the business community seeks out attractive people to fill available positions, because *looks sell*. Automobile, cosmetic, and apparel manufactures have long recognized this fact of human nature. Those who have the responsibility of hiring new employees confirm that—when all other qualifications are equal—a pleasing appearance gives an applicant (or a candidate for promotion) the advantage over competitors who choose to ignore the advantage that investing in a more pleasing appearance would give them.

The *Journal of Personality and Social Psychology* reports that although definitions of beauty have varied through the ages, the fact that favors are granted to individuals considered handsome or beautiful has never changed. But the granting of such "favors" goes farther back in history than the modern medical literature. Aristotle wrote, "Beauty is a better recommendation than any letter of introduction."

Let's pause here to examine Aristotle's venerable admonition. In the statement I shared above, this brilliant Greek philosopher, recognized as one of the greatest minds in history, was saying, "The way you look when you enter the room for an interview establishes an immediate and indelible impression in the mind of the interviewer." If that impression is positive, you are already ahead of the competitors who entered the room ahead of you or some that might follow. Then you can build upon that impression.

Otherwise, you begin your quest for success behind the others competing for the same position. Can you *overcome* the negative first impression you created by a less than ideal appearance? The realistic answer is yes; it is possible. However, why count on Big Brother laws that pertain to political correctness? Why not present your best self at the outset? Why would you not give yourself the best opportunity to appeal to the inherent—and indisputable—nature of our species?

Given the current politically correct environment, these are questions many books on dream achievement shy away from addressing.

Is it any wonder that individuals who choose to undergo appearance-enhancing procedures do so for economic reasons—as an investment in themselves and the welfare of those who depend upon them? A pleasing appearance is an advantage not only for the fashion model, television and movie personality, corporate executive, professional, or sales person but for anyone whose work or lifestyle requires interaction with the public—the ultimate consumer of goods, products, and services. It is a world in which every job applicant or individual seeking health, happiness, and prosperity is forced to compete.

Educators have shared with me that the young people they teach relate better to them when they put forth the effort to look their best. A pleasing appearance offers other advantages. Renowned psychologist Dr. Perry Buffington reported that for students, "good looks affect school grades." Furthermore, according to Dr. Buffington, one's looks also "determine who will become our friends and shortens stays in mental hospitals."[3] Each of these factors increases a person's chances to become prosperous, in whatever way they define prosperity.

No Longer Just for the Rich and Famous

People in the upper socioeconomic brackets are not the only ones who undergo appearance-enhancing procedures; working people living out

---

3. Perry W. Buffington, *Your Behavior Is Showing: Forty Prescriptions for Understanding and Liking Yourself* (Nashville: Hillbrook House, 1988).

their lives on a budget do too. Most people plan for their appearance-enhancing procedures like they plan for a vacation, a new addition to their home, a swimming pool, or a new automobile. Based upon indisputable evidence, they accept an enhanced appearance as an investment in themselves.

Today, financing opportunities are available for everyone, regardless of their income. As a result, people from all walks of life are taking advantage of creative ways to put forward a more impressive appearance in what I prefer to refer to as the "marketplace of human competition." When people look better, their pride and ego are bolstered, and—surprisingly enough—it has been shown that when people feel good about themselves, they perform better and are compensated accordingly. I received the following letter from a young woman who underwent an enhancement procedure to her nose. It affirms the statements above:

> Dr. McCollough,
> Before my rhinoplasty, I was always cautious about the way I positioned myself in a room, making sure that no one ever caught a glimpse of my profile. I was a freshman in college and didn't involve myself in many on campus activities because having to constantly be aware of my nose was exhausting.
>
> I am happy to report that following my surgery I rushed for sorority and graduated with Honors . . . I gained many friends and was involved in many on campus clubs and intramural activities.
>
> Whereas before, I always felt timid when working with patients, following the surgery I got a job in a dental clinic which helped prepare me for where I am today.

Corporate America certainly understands the value Americans place upon personal appearance. Billions of dollars are spent each year by people from all walks of life on nonsurgical measures such as cosmetics, accessories, fashionable wardrobes, vitamins, health foods, and weight-control products. Many of these same individuals *also* undergo plastic surgery and take extraordinary care of their skin, hair, and nails. These same women and men tend to coordinate their wardrobes and pay attention to their weight.

Cosmetic (or aesthetic) plastic surgery can often improve your appearance by bringing into harmony unsightly facial and body features or by eliminating some of the conspicuous external indications associated with the aging process. Reconstructive plastic surgery, on the other hand, attempts to restore portions of your body to the state in which they might have existed prior to an injury, infection, tumor removal, or previously unsuccessful surgery. The correction of many congenital defects (birth defects) also falls under this category.

Aesthetic skin care encompasses a variety of methods designed to improve the quality, texture, and health of one's skin. Medical aestheticians can also serve as consultants for scientific skin care, professionally recommended makeup, skin cancer prevention, improved toning of the muscles of the face and neck, and some medical skin conditions, such as acne, age spots, and precancerous blemishes. Personal fitness and nutritional counselors also play an important role in health and well-being.

Irrefutably, the world in which we live is a highly competitive place. Those who thrive in such an environment understand not only how to survive but how to rise above the masses and thrive in challenging circumstances. If you have decided to give yourself the best chance to succeed in the world and have not yet discovered ways to do so, this book provides answers.

Everything in Moderation

We have all seen fellow human beings who've gone beyond the reasonable and natural when it comes to altering their appearance and body. As a general rule, any alteration taken to the extreme will usually be viewed by the discerning eye as *unattractive*. The best policy is to exercise balance and good taste in all things.

CHAPTER 5

How Old Are You?

Not that long ago, a woman came to me for a consultation. She was interested in age-reversing surgery. After the usual salutations, she asked me, "How old do you think I am?"

I responded with a truthful answer: "Ma'am, I don't know how old you are; nor does it matter. I know that somewhere on the forms you filled out prior to our visit, your birthday is recorded; however, I never look at that part of the form. I am much more concerned with how old your body actually is and the current state of your health."

Taken aback by my answer, she said again, "How old do you think I am?"

I replied, "As long as your doctor tells me that you are healthy enough to undergo a twilight anesthesia and the procedures I will recommend for you, your age is irrelevant."

Still insistent on discussing her age, she volunteered, "I am eighty-six years old. I am self-sufficient and drive back and forth from Alabama to Arkansas every month to visit my great-grandchildren. All the members of my family lived well into their nineties, and I expect to surpass them."

The "rest of the story," as the venerable Paul Harvey was famous for telling, is this: the woman's doctors cleared her for a face and eyelid lift, and she came through the surgery like a champ.

A couple of months later, she returned for a routine postoperative visit and brought with her a gentleman I had not previously met. She introduced the gentleman as her fiancé. She proceeded to inform me that her fiancé was in his late sixties and that she was in her mideighties. She went even further by bringing attention to the fact that, following the surgery I had performed, she looked younger than he did and, because of his health issues, would probably outlive him.

The facts were the facts. She was correct in her assessment of the situation at hand. I share this story to emphasize a fact of life. Every individual has two "ages": a chronological one and a biological one. Your chronological age is determined by how many years you've lived. Your biological age is a reflection of how old your body actually is and how old it appears to an observer.

When it comes to the overall health and appearance of your body, a positive outlook on life cannot be underestimated. People who look for the good and positive in every situation tend to find whatever it is they seek. The opposite is also true. People who look for the bad and ugly in the world around them tend to find it.

Let's step aside from age-reversing surgery for a minute to address the biological aspects of the aging process. Balanced nutrition (with appropriate supplementation) is also a major factor in remaining healthy and attractive, as is physical activity that keeps circulation flowing and muscles strong. Weight-bearing exercise also tends to keep bones strong by combating osteoporosis, an often overlooked risk factor for men and women over the age of sixty. Balance issues also increase with age, and 90 percent of individuals over the age of seventy who have advanced osteoporosis and break a hip from a fall die within a year, often from related complications. Unsteadiness and fractures of brittle bones are often the onset of the downhill spiral.

Maintaining balance with your body's hormonal system is also crucial to good health and a pleasing appearance, as I address in the next chapter.

CHAPTER 6

Beyond the Surface

A few years back, a patient consulted me for a second opinion about her face. Just a few months before, she had undergone a full facelift with blepharoplasty (upper and lower eyelid rejuvenation).

Because her initial surgery did not achieve the desired results, her original surgeon had agreed to perform additional surgery. Upon examining her, I noticed that the tissues around her eyes were puffy and that her skin was dry and wrinkled, not only on her face but on her arms and hands.

Immediately, I took off my surgeon's hat and put on my doctor's hat—my metaphysician's hat. I called upon the training I had received from medical school, my internship, and the countless hours and nights I'd spent caring for patients in outlying emergency rooms and nursing homes. I asked questions about this patient's overall health. By answering only two or three targeted questions, the patient gave me what I needed. However, in order to confirm my suspicions, I ordered a series of laboratory tests. The results of the tests confirmed my working diagnosis: her body was deficient in thyroid hormone. This, I concluded, was why her facial tissues were puffy, why her skin was dry and scaly, why her wrinkles were so deep, and why she felt tired and cold when others in the same room with her did not.

With a diagnosis in hand, I referred this woman to a colleague who specialized in hormone-replacement therapy. The photographs below demonstrate the improvement in her appearance with nothing but thyroid replacement therapy. No surgical or skin-rejuvenation procedures were performed.

Almost miraculously, her pretreatment symptoms of fatigue, weakness, intolerance to cold air and weather, forgetfulness, and fluid retention, as well as her troublesome dry skin and puffy face, disappeared—thereby lifting her spirits and her life.

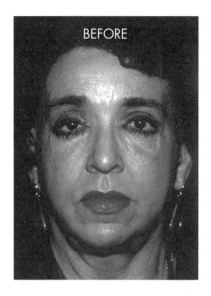
BEFORE

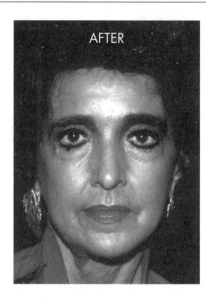
AFTER

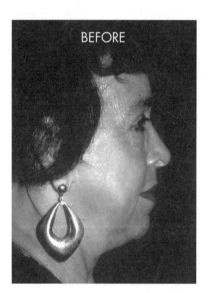
BEFORE

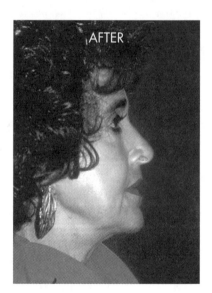
AFTER

Only thyroid replacement therapy.

The enhancement in this woman's appearance and life was no miracle. It was the result of lessons learned from my endocrinology professors in medical school—particularly Dr. Clifton Meador—before I became an appearance-enhancement surgeon. I offer this story as a tribute to Dr. Meador and as a reminder that unhealthy conditions on the inside are expressed on the outside and must be considered prior to embarking upon surgical treatments.

After her medical condition was corrected, additional procedures could have added to this patient's comprehensive enhancement program. She could have benefitted from a skin-resurfacing procedure to further improve the wrinkling around her eyes. She could also have had the drooping appearance of her lower eyelids corrected. However, she chose to accept the improvement she had obtained and move forward. I was fine with that. After all, my responsibility as a metaphysician and surgeon was to help this woman enhance the quality of her life, with or without additional surgery.

My takeaway message is this: although surgery might need to be included in your comprehensive appearance-enhancement plan, other factors must be considered. To paraphrase an age-old proverb, there is a "time for everything." However, when it comes to enhancing your health and appearance, there is a time to seek second opinions and to make sure that the procedures and products recommended to you—even those suggested by physicians and surgeons with celebrated reputations—are the ones that are right for the current time and underlying circumstances of your life. But how are you to know which so-called experts to trust? As experts deliver advice, pay close attention to their body language. Look into their eyes and see if you perceive honesty and integrity. Listen between the lines of what they are saying to you for a genuine regard for *your* welfare. If any of those factors are not clearly identified, keep searching until you find the right professional *for you*. When it comes to your welfare (or that of those who rely upon you for advice and counsel), never allow yourself to be pressured into making a decision that could affect your life . . . for whatever is left of it.

With those thoughts in mind, let's look at some of the nonsurgical measures you might want to consider on your way toward becoming the best you possible. In future chapters, I'll address a wide variety of surgical and nonsurgical options.

Very early in my life, I came to grips with my "place in the universe." As the son of a small-town plumber, I realized that my place lay beyond seeing that an ample supply of fresh water entered peoples' homes and not-so-fresh water entered the sewage systems of their communities. Not until I'd obtained all the education that my mother and father had dreamed of for me did I come to realize that the word "water" could be substituted for the words "knowledge" and "wisdom."

As a young physician and surgeon, I chose to devote my professional life to enhancing the life experiences of my fellow human beings by bringing fresh and pure ideas to their minds and bodies while finding ways to eliminate corruptive ideas and send them into the sewers of human thought. For this mission, I will forever give credit to my parents. It is one from which I have never veered and never will.

In this book, I've attempted to share ways that, if followed, can assist you in the process of enhancing all three components of your being: your mind, body, and spirit.

Because your skin is the most visible element of your body—and its largest organ—I will elaborate on the case history I introduced at the beginning of this chapter. While the wrinkled and puffy skin of her face drove her to consulting with me, deeper issues were lurking silently inside—hormonal issues. My responsibility was to recognize those issues and refer her to a colleague for treatment.

The Skin: A Barrier, Organ, and Factory

A fact not generally known beyond the appearance- and health-enhancement professions is that the skin protects the inside of the human body against harmful bacteria, viruses, and chemicals. It is also the largest organ of the human body and a manufacturer of an essential vitamin—vitamin D.

As was the woman's case referenced in this chapter, your skin is also one of the earliest indicators that the biological systems designed to keep you well could be out of balance. Rather than simply treating the visible signs of aging, metaphysicians and surgeons provide skin therapies that are designed not only to make the skin look better but to help address the underlying conditions that the appearance of unhealthy skin heralds—the most common of which are years of unprotected sun and wind exposure. Unbalanced hormones and poor dietary choices follow closely behind. In future chapters, we will examine these correctable factors.

Nonsurgical Rejuvenation Procedures

A variety of nonsurgical procedures and products assist in camouflaging—but not correcting—the signs of aging that are exhibited by the outside skin. However, comprehensive rejuvenation professionals serve as more than a prescription center or filling station for commercially created, topically applied products, injectable fillers, and muscle-paralyzing agents. Elite Rejuvenology centers fill a long-overdue void in the appearance- and health-enhancement industry by serving as comprehensive age-inhibition and lifestyle-management resources.

The professionally prescribed and overseen skin-care programs and products offered by elite Rejuvenology centers can give your skin a more youthful appearance, but only on a temporary basis. Medical-grade injectable fillers also provide short-term improvement of wrinkles and creases caused by aging. However, you might be looking for therapies that are more effective and less costly in the long run. If so, you might dream of being as healthy as you look, and you might want to look your best longer than some of the most widely promoted and temporary therapies can allow.

Are you seeking more permanent eradication of deep facial lines, grooves, and thinning lips? If so, your own collagen can be inserted through tiny incisions by an aesthetic surgeon duly trained in the technique. It is a technique that I have more than twenty years' experience in performing, with a high degree of success, and it's now offered by many of the appearance-enhancing surgeons I have personally trained, as well as by those who have attended my lectures and read the articles I have published in peer-reviewed journals and chapters in textbooks.

Muscle-paralyzing neurotoxins such as Botox and Dysport minimize the kinds of wrinkling and scowling that occur with frequent and exaggerated facial expressions, but, again, only on a temporary basis. For best results, retreatment every several months is required. I emphasize that neurotoxins correct only wrinkles that occur when your facial muscles are called into action. Wrinkles that are present when your face is at rest require one of the skin-resurfacing procedures I'll address later in this chapter.

Other nonsurgical or minimally invasive therapies designed to rejuvenate the skin of the face and neck include level 2 dermabrasion, chemical peels, fractioned laser treatments, and (to a lesser extent) microneedling with radiofrequency. Level 1 procedures such as microdermabrasion, intense pulse light (IPL), and epidermal chemical peels may address the desires of someone looking for a short-term solution for an important event in their lives, such as a class reunion, wedding, bar or bat mitzvah, or graduation.

Level 1 laser therapy, superficial (epidermal) chemical peels, and microdermabrasion procedures are performed by Rejuvenology physicians and surgeons and, in some states, by physician extenders (physician assistants, nurse practitioners, registered nurses, and aestheticians). These superficial technologies exfoliate the dull, scaly skin that collects on the surface as new skin is constantly being created underneath. With Level 1 exfoliating procedures and products, your skin will exhibit a younger, healthier glow and smoother texture, but only temporarily. These treatments must be repeated on a monthly basis.

For level 2 and 3 conditions, such as deeper wrinkles and precancerous or deeply pigmented spots, more invasive epidermal *and* dermal therapies are required and provide long-lasting results. I'll address these treatment alternatives in future chapters and explain why they tend to provide more visible—and longer-lasting—results.

CHAPTER 7

Nonsurgical Skin-Enhancement Products:

Help or Hype?

A wide variety of skin-care products are available on the nonprescription market. I'm sorry to disappoint you and millions of your fellow appearance-enhancement seekers by revealing that many of these nonprescription products, some of which misleadingly represent themselves as "facelifts in a bottle," offer more *hype* than *help*. Anything available in a bottle—or without a prescription from a licensed physician—is incapable of removing inches of loose, sagging, wrinkled, and sun-damaged skin. The vast majority of commercially available products that minimize wrinkles do just that—minimize them, and only for a few hours or days at best.

It is with your best interest in mind that I include two venerable admonitions that apply to nonphysician-delivered remedies for the ever-mounting aging process. First: *if it sounds too good to be true, it usually is too good to be true.* The second admonition is one that I feel sure you have heard before: *buyer beware!* As an author, metaphysician, and appearance-enhancing surgeon sworn to the Hippocratic Oath, I view it as my responsibility to share with you a lifetime of experience relating to the appearance- and health-enhancement professions. Most of all, I consider it my responsibility to share with you the truth as I have come to know it during the four-plus decades I have devoted my professional life to caring for more than twenty-five thousand patients.

In addition to being a board-certified facial plastic surgeon, I also identify as a clinical Rejuvenologist. A Rejuvenologist is a medical professional who incorporates into their patient-care protocols the arts and sciences required to rejuvenate the human mind, body, and spirit. This means that I take it upon myself to try to recapture the state of youth and vitality that once existed in each of my patients, even if doing so dictates that I refer them to a health-care professional more capable of dealing with their conditions than I am.

I once served as president of the International Council of Integrative Medicine. "Integrative medicine" refers to incorporating the procedures and processes of every necessary branch of the health-care industry into the comprehensive care of each individual patient.

Although I was not introduced to the integrative care of a given patient during my traditional medical training, I owe this expanded scope of my ability to care for my patients to the late Dr. Brian Costello, an integrative psychologist and colleague from Australia who wrote the foreword to my book *Let Us Make Man*. Because of Dr. Costello's influence upon my integrative approach to life enhancement, I feel it a duty to address the often overused term "facelift." As I was taught and have observed for more than four decades, when it comes to facial rejuvenation, the term "facelift" implies that multiple layers of the face and neck (the skin, muscle, and sagging fat) are surgically repositioned and secured into a state of existence that preceded the onset of the ravaging signs of aging every one of us exhibits. In an authentic "facelift," only *after* the deeper structures (the muscles and fat of the face and neck) are addressed is excess and age-ravaged skin removed and then discarded. The takeaway fact from this descriptive overview of the operation is that unless the underlying structures are supported, tightening the sagging skin of your face will be short lived, for it is a proven fact of medical science that skin placed under tension will stretch. The best example, with which most women can identify, is that during pregnancy, the skin of your abdomen stretches to accommodate the expanding mass of your baby underneath. I also take advantage of this fact when repairing defects that resulted from the removal of skin cancer.

In short, for a product or procedure to qualify as a "facelift," more than the superficial layers of facial and neck skin must be addressed—and in a manner that complies with the rules of anatomical logic and surgical common sense. There is one exception to this rule. Level 3 chemical peels that are performed by a licensed physician and require two to three weeks to heal will, in fact, tighten and lift the skin of the lower face and neck, albeit to a lesser degree than a face-lift. In my experience, lasers are not as effective in doing so.

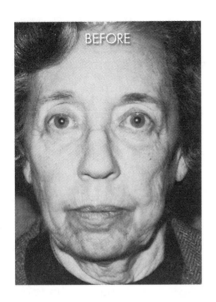
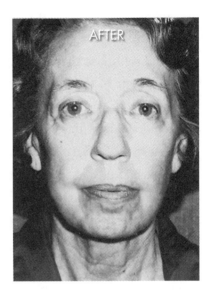

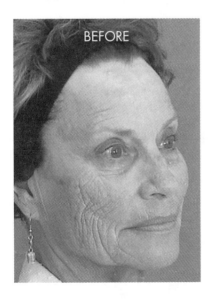
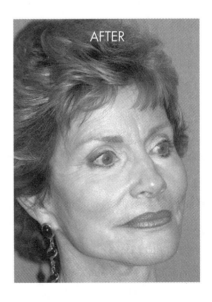

The preceding notwithstanding, among the plethora of commercial products and "minimally invasive" procedures available, a select few have been determined (through research and experience) to be helpful in giving human skin a more youthful appearance. This includes those that contain higher concentrations of Retin-A, which (in most states) require a prescription from a licensed physician—and for good reason. If you choose to use these products, insist that you be prescribed lower concentrations of the product to begin with in order to give your skin an opportunity to adapt to the higher concentrations that might be prescribed at a later date.

It is a scientific fact that products prescribed by Rejuvenology-focused physicians and physician extenders and administered with ongoing professional oversight tend to be more effective and provide happier outcomes and fewer complications, not only for the client but for the provider.

A fact little known to the average consumer is that the reason some medications and preparations are available "over the counter" or in many nonphysician-operated spas is that the concentration and combinations of active ingredients in those medications are considerably lower, and therefore less effective, than in those administered or prescribed by a physician. In addition, products prescribed and provided from physicians' offices must be manufactured to higher specifications and oversight. It's another example of the age-old principle that the consumer usually gets what they pay for.

Here, I interject another "buyer beware" admonition. Just because a physician *endorses* a product or procedure does not mean that the product or procedure has been subjected to scientific scrutiny. In the medical profession, the level a procedure or product is required to meet is known as evidence-based medicine and surgery. This means that the product has undergone unbiased research that was conducted on a large number of patients by someone who had no personal or financial interest in the outcome of the data collected.

The takeaway message here is this: consumers and medical colleagues alike are obliged to check out not only the product or device promoted but also its promoter. As a consumer, you should ask your provider whether they have any financial interest in the company that manufactures or distributes the product recommended to you. You have a right to know.

It is also important that you are not misled by the overused term "natural." A number of "natural" products are harmful to the human body, including marijuana, tobacco, and products that derive from the poppy plant (cocaine, heroin, etc.).

In keeping with the "buyer beware" admonition, when it comes to your health and appearance, I suggest you become your own best advocate. Ask the hard questions, and do not settle for answers that your mind tells you to investigate further.

As that advice applies to age-defying products and procedures, I should also emphasize that longer-lasting results are obtained when the professionals providing nonsurgical procedures and products work hand in hand with integrative Rejuvenology physicians and surgeons and vice versa.

In your search for an enhanced appearance and the documented advantages that go with it, how are you to know whom to trust? The best answer I can offer is that it's your body, mind, health, and happiness at stake. You owe it to yourself to invest the time of doing the necessary research. Investigate the training, experience, and professional reputation of each provider under consideration. Take nothing for granted. And keep in mind that while certificates and certifications should be considered, *experience counts*. And lots of experience counts big time. With each of the procedures that you are considering, demand to see before and after results of procedures personally performed by the doctor or therapist you are consulting. If you detect any hesitation in your demands, scratch that professional off your list of candidates.

When you decide to change the way you look, feel, and perform, you are giving yourself a gift that could pay huge dividends and help you to become the person of your dreams. Take the time to personally interview professionals whose reputations have stood the test of time and see if your concerns and their recommendations are compatible. Ask the hard questions. Listen between the lines, and read between the words. The list of inquires below is a good place to start.

- How many procedures of the type we are discussing have you *personally* performed?
- For how many years have you been performing the procedures that you are recommending for me?
- Setting aside short-term results, what are your long-term experiences?
- Have you performed—or recommended—the procedures you are recommending for me on a family member?
- Who will actually be performing the procedures being discussed, and who will be monitoring my healing and recovery process, not only during the hours shortly thereafter but during the following days, weeks, and months? Who will manage—and correct—any problems or complications that might ensue?
- How will the costs of future treatments (should they become necessary) be shared?

While the questions above might appear to be confrontational in nature, as a consumer and body owner, you deserve straightforward answers to each of them. It is your body, and you are entitled to know the pros and cons of any treatment initiative to which you consent. In fact, reputable physicians will also comment on areas of your face and body that are not ready for any treatment. For the areas that are ready for treatment, doctors and physician extenders will offer a document that asks you (the recipient of treatment) to consent (give written permission) to the treatment recommended.

Medical providers are held to a standard of care that includes informing their patients of alternative methods of treating any condition under consideration. If your doctor or provider did not discuss or provide in writing other ways of addressing your concerns, you have not been duly informed, and the provider might not have met the standard required by law. Furthermore, if printed materials are provided, *be sure to read them*, for many consent forms include a section in which you attest that you have read the materials offered prior to treatment. If your questions are not answered, do not sign the form until they are.

As a provider of medical and surgical care for more than four decades, I recommend that you do not just glibly sign any document presented to you, especially when it comes to your health and well-being. Read it, and if you are not fully comfortable with what you are about to sign, simply say, "I'd like to take this home with me, mull it over, and seek counsel if I have any questions." If the physician or assistant is hesitant or offended when you speak those words, that reaction should be an indication that you should seek further consultation. Succumbing to "hard sell" or "special offer" tactics often results in disappointment or worse.

Inside-Out Care

As previously noted, the way your skin appears is an indicator of a wide variety of conditions that exist beneath it. Undiagnosed medical conditions (hormone imbalances, thyroid deficiencies, collagen disorders, poor nutrition, age-progressing stress, grief, or potentially life-threatening cancerous conditions) are often reflected in the appearance and texture of your skin. This might be the best argument for why you should develop a professional relationship with a skin-care provider who is either a physician or closely affiliated with a physician's clinic that abides by a quality standard of care.

For these reasons, professionally administered appearance enhancement—such as skin care or management of nutrition, weight, or age—should be approached from inside out *and* outside in. From a sample of your blood, physicians can determine whether a variety of hormones are out of balance, whether you need to supplement your diet, or whether there is any indication of a biologic imbalance of your internal organ systems. If scientific testing shows that you have an imbalance, a physician who is focused on caring for the mind, body, and spirit can recommend the appropriate corrective measures. In some cases, however, referral to your personal physician or a condition-specific medical specialist might be indicated.

As I see it, a Rejuvenologist is not always the professional who can treat every unhealthy condition. Rather, they are a health-care professional who accepts the responsibility of seeing that patients are placed under the care of the most qualified professional or team of professionals. It could be said that a Rejuvenologist is a gatekeeper to comprehensive enhancement of health and appearance.

If you are willing to do the things that are required to look your best—the things I share with you throughout this book—you are likely to find better health even if finding better health was not your primary objective. In the next chapter, I address something that has plagued many of us: maintaining a healthy weight.

CHAPTER 8

The Weight Factor

Obesity, as much as any other condition I address in this book, affects the mind, body, and spirit. The condition appears to originate not from our stomachs but from within the thought centers of our minds; therefore, the more you know about the condition, the better equipped you will be to remain in control of your weight. The truth is that except in extreme situations, we choose to be fat—or not. How can I make such a statement? Because there was a time in my own life when I experienced being fat firsthand.

At the age of twelve and a height of five feet, I weighed nearly thirty pounds more than I should have. I played Little League baseball, but I was unable to wear the full uniform worn by my fellow teammates. I played in "husky" (meaning plus-sized) blue jeans. I was able to wear the shirt portion of the uniform, with my number on the back, but could only button the top two buttons. That meant that I had to wear a T-shirt underneath. Because of the excess weight I carried, it would be an understatement to say that I could not run very fast. In fact, the laughter coming from the stands when I ran down the first-base line still reverberates in my mind.

Because I never expected to be an athlete, I took up the trumpet and played in my high school's band. I recall an afternoon during band practice when a photographer came to the stadium and took a photograph for the school annual. A few months later, the annual was published. As I thumbed through it, I found the photograph of our relatively small (in numbers) marching band, the one that the photographer had snapped on that fall afternoon. However, as I studied the photograph, I was unable to find myself in the picture. I vividly recalled the names of the two band members I'd stood between in formation. As I readily identified them, I suddenly realized that the overweight person who stood between them—the one I did not recognize—was *me!* Until that day, I had never seen a full-body photograph of myself. The mirror I dressed before each day reflected only the upper third of my body. At that moment, I realized just how overweight I was and why the girls in my class had more interest in dating other boys. On that revelatory day, I recognized the problem and made a pledge that I would never again be fat.

A drastic reduction in the number of calories I ingested, coupled with running (rather than riding) to and from school (which was located across town from my home) each day, did the trick. Over the next three months, I lost the excess pounds I had been carrying and—at the same time—began to grow taller.

In the 1950s, dieting was more difficult, as diet foods and drinks were not available in grocery stores. However, when a family friend heard that I was trying to lose weight, she gave my mother a recipe for a diet milkshake. I recall that the shake was made with raw eggs and condensed milk. It proved to be the dietary crutch I needed.

A few months later, I not only was able to fit into regular clothes but began to see my classmates look at me in a different light. I felt better about myself. My confidence in pursuing other challenges and relationships was bolstered. Having lost the weight, it was up to me to keep it off. I liked the new me and pledged to never again be fat.

I laid down my trumpet and turned instead to sports. Each spring, I put on the uniform of my high school's baseball team. This time, the

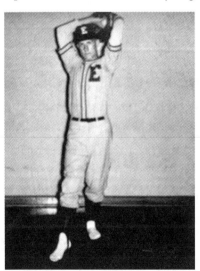

top and bottom of the uniform both fit perfectly—and so did the football and basketball uniforms I proudly wore during games with fans in the stands.

A few years later, I was given the opportunity to play for one of the greatest college football coaches in America: Coach Paul W. "Bear" Bryant. My senior year at the University of Alabama, I played on a national championship team and received all-American honors. Shortly thereafter, I was drafted by the Dallas Cowboys. The rest of the story is beyond the scope of this book, but suffice to say that returning to a reasonable and healthy weight opened doors that previously had been closed.

I still battle with maintaining a weight that fits my age and height. That fat thirteen-year-old trumpet player standing in the middle of Enterprise High School's football field, practicing for halftime show on an upcoming Friday night in the fall of 1956, is ever present in my mind. Some six decades later, that mental picture is all the deterrent I need to keep from having to buy larger clothes. In fact, at the time of this writing, my weight is the same as when I graduated college. Mind you, some of that weight has shifted a bit. However, it is nice to see my scale each morning register a weight that makes me feel better about myself.

Admittedly, there have been times when I lost focus and let my weight get a bit out of control. As a result, my clothes began to fit more snugly than felt comfortable—physically and mentally. But rather than buying a new wardrobe, I refocused and chose to lose the weight.

So when I offer advice on weight management, I do so with the voice of experience. Although I could write an entire chapter about my experience of being fat, suffice to say the following: as a person who has been fat and then has not been, I can say that, at least for me, not being fat has proven to be the better choice.

Obesity Defined

Before I go any further, it might be helpful to define obesity. The Obesity Medicine Association (OMA) defines it as "a chronic, relapsing, multifactorial, neurobehavioral disease, wherein an increase in body fat promotes adipose tissue dysfunction and abnormal fat mass physical forces, resulting in adverse metabolic, biomechanical, and psychosocial health consequences."[4] The Centers for Disease Control and Prevention

---

4. Anna Welcome, "Definition of Obesity," Obesity Medicine Association, August 29, 2017, https:// obesitymedicine.org/definition-of-obesity/.

(CDC) provides a somewhat extended definition: "weight that is higher than what is considered as a healthy weight for a given height."[5] Other organizations get more technical and relate it to body mass index (BMI). For the sake of this discussion, I choose to keep it rather simple and use the OMA's definition. It addresses the behavioral and psychological parts of the condition.

Here's a fact that is likely to surprise you: even though great strides have been made in combating conditions that rob victims of health, happiness, and longevity, obesity still remains one of the most common *treatable* unhealthy conditions in the United States.

A more disturbing fact is that the children being born in our country today are the first generation in more than a century with a shorter life expectancy than their parents. This is mostly a result of the obesity epidemic and is a sad statement about the lack of self-discipline that is permeating our society.

Being overweight not only detracts from our appearance but has a negative impact on our health. We are much more likely to have high blood pressure and type 2 diabetes if we are overweight. Because of the weight we are carrying around, we are more likely to suffer from back and knee problems. And it appears that obesity is related to the development of cancer. In addition, when we gain weight, the skin that envelopes the structures of our face and body is stretched, making it even more susceptible to the sags, bulges, and wrinkles that telegraph aging.

If you choose to lose weight, it will be necessary to force your metabolism into what amounts to a starvation mode, which often causes your skin to appear malnourished. This is where scientific micronutrient testing can be helpful. Because you have driven your body into relative starvation, vitamin and mineral supplementation might be indicated. This is a mere smattering of the scientific research and personal experience I

5. "Defining Adult Overweight and Obesity," Centers for Disease Control and Prevention, last reviewed April 11, 2017, https://www.cdc.gov/obesity/adult/defining.html.

want to share with you here—as motivation, I hope, to get your attention, as that early photograph of myself got mine.

While returning to a more ideal weight is beneficial to the health of internal organs, roller-coaster dieting—defined by massive weight swings—will compromise your skin's elasticity. Regardless of the stimulus, stretching human skin leads to sags and droops over the entire body, some of which can become permanent, especially beyond menopause (in women) and andropause (in men), the biological age at which the sex hormones begin to shut down.

If you are a woman, you might find it difficult to maintain your weight following menopause. If you are a man, you might experience similar difficulties as you progress through andropause. Part of the issue is the change in your body's levels of sex hormones (estrogen and testosterone). Scientific testing allows your physician to balance those hormones and offset many of the conditions traditionally identified with menopause or andropause. Keep the thyroid factor in mind as well. Lower-than-normal levels of thyroid hormone can cause weight gain via two ways: excessive accumulation of swelling in the body's tissues and lower-than-normal metabolism of foods.

Women who have experienced stretching of the skin of the abdomen during pregnancy can attest to the fact that "stretch marks" rarely, if ever, disappear. In severe cases, surgical excision for the stretch marks lower in the abdomen can be achieved with a "tummy tuck" (abdominoplasty). (See chapter 30.)

The hard—yet encouraging—fact about weight management is that outside of hormonal factors, managing your weight is not nearly as complicated as you might think. It is simply a matter of discipline—exercising the free will given to you at the time of your creation. Choose to limit the amount and kinds of food taken into your body on a daily basis. Managing your weight is also a matter of keeping score—that is, exercising the self-discipline to balance the number of calories ingested each day with the number of calories expended through physical activity.

It goes without saying that the more physical activity you engage in, the more calories you will burn. But for most people, burning calories through exercise alone is not the answer to weight management. For example, you must walk a mile at a rapid pace to burn the number of calories taken in with two cookies, a nondietetic beverage, half a medium-sized bag of popcorn, or small piece of cake or pie.

Because it can be confusing, let's take a moment here to better understand the term *calorie*. It is a scientific reference to the amount of energy required to raise the temperature of a flask of water. In nutritional circles, it is a way to measure the energy value of foods (carbohydrates, proteins, and fats). Said another way, foods or drinks that contain one hundred calories will supply one hundred calories of energy for the individual who ingests them—the amount of energy required for an individual who weighs one hundred pounds to walk a mile on level ground at a normal pace. Unused calories are converted to fatty acids, which are then stored inside the expandable walls of fat cells located throughout the body. As a result, the fat cells expand and occupy more space beneath the individual's skin.

In reality, a fat cell is a tiny balloon—a microscopic storage container—filled with oil (fatty acids). As a medical student, I was taught that each of us is born with a certain number of fat cells in our body, determined by the genes we inherit from our parents. Except when liposuction or some other process that removes or ruptures fat cells is carried out, the number of fat cells in the body remains constant throughout life. Each cell simply expands as unused calories are converted to fatty acids.

All diet plans (human or otherwise) are based upon forcing a body into a state of starvation. The 600 or so calories stored in the liver are the first source of calories used up during periods of starvation (or what is known as: a *catabolic* state of existence, or self-cannibalization). Fatty acids are the second source of calories, and muscle is the third. Muscle is not broken down into calories until fat cells throughout the body have been cannibalized. At the stage of muscle cannibalism, life becomes precarious. (More on this process later in this chapter).

During lectures on nutrition and metabolism in medical school, my physiology and biochemistry professors used the following example. The body of an "average woman" weighing 120 pounds burns approximately 1,600 calories per day, *without* a strenuous exercise routine. The body of an "average man" weighing approximately 180 to 200 pounds burns between 1,800 and 2,000 calories per day. So, if the average woman does not ingest more than 1,600 calories per day, she should maintain a relatively stable weight. If the average man does not ingest more than 1,800 to 2,000 calories per day, he should maintain his current weight. When exercise is added to the equation, every mile walked or run offsets 100 ingested calories. I hope you are seeing that weight management is a matter of simple math—calories ingested versus calories burned—and that the entire process is controlled from within your mind!

Admittedly, during the past several decades, the size and weight of human beings have evolved. Both men and women tend to be taller and weigh more than our "average" counterparts did before the turn of the twenty-first century. Among the settlers who migrated to America in the 1600s and 1700s, the average height of a man was five feet two inches. The average height of a woman was two inches shorter. Two hundred years later, the average heights of both men and women have increased by several inches and are increasing further with every passing decade.

As the average height increases, the average weight has also become greater. Even so, the ideal proportions of our bodies as described by Leonardo da Vinci have not changed, except through our own lack of self-discipline. This is a fact that many of us would rather not face.

If, however, *gaining* weight is your objective, you must ingest more calories than you burn through

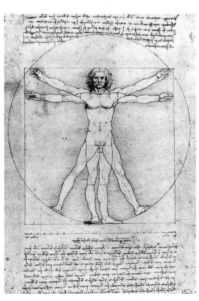

physical activity every day. In my opinion, commercially available products that claim to "burn belly fat" are more hype than help. When examined under a microscope, belly fat is no different than fat in the remainder of your body, so the idea that a product attacks belly fat more than it does any other fat cell has no scientific basis.

Thyroid-replacement medications will speed up one's metabolism and can affect one's weight. Many other weight-loss products and medications contain caffeine, theobromine (found in tea), or some other medication or herb that will increase your heart rate and raise your blood pressure. Keep in mind that every medication has side effects, some of which could be more damaging than the condition being treated.

The reality is that weight management is similar to balancing your checking account: calories *in* versus calories *out*; calories *burned* versus calories *consumed*.

Many commercial diet plans, especially those that provide the foods you are instructed to eat each day, do the calorie-counting exercise for you. Truth is, if followed, all commercial diet plans can be effective in the short term. However, unless you are committed to purchasing meals from that company for life and eating or drinking nothing else, maintaining your weight becomes a challenge. In fact, the statistics are shocking. Ninety-five percent of those who lose weight on a given commercial plan tend to gain all the weight back—plus some. Entertainer Marie Osmond appears to be the exception. For best results and a lifetime of looking and being thinner and more fit, you—and those you care for and about—would be wise to consult with a trained health professional and learn how to manage your weight with food sources available at grocery stores, fresh food markets, and restaurants. A growing number of restaurants list on their menus the total calories contained in each dish.

Let's examine a long-recognized "secret" to weight management that many commercial diet plans choose not to address. The secret is actually no secret; rather, it is a matter of simple math. I call it the Calorie-Counting Solution for Weight Management (TCCS). It is based upon a simple equation I have already shared with you: calories in versus calories expended (or burned).

Here's how the math works. If you eliminate just one hundred calories per day (by avoiding ingesting them or by burning them through physical activity), at the end of thirty days, you will have eliminated three thousand calories from your total caloric intake. Your body is designed with such precision that it will harvest the calories it needs from somewhere within itself, at least for as long as the supply lasts. The vast number of calories stored within your body exists in fat cells in the form of fatty acids. Three thousand calories are contained in one pound of fat. Let me repeat that: three thousand calories are contained in one pound of fat. So, burn three thousand calories more than you take in during any given time frame, and you will lose one pound.

When physical activity is added to the process, weight loss moves ahead on a more rapid basis. In its simplest form, the math equation for TCCS is "pounds lost per month = days in the month times net calories eliminated per day (in multiples of 100)." Say every month lasts thirty days. Since one pound of fat contains 3,000 calories, you will lose one pound over the course of a month when you eliminate 100 calories per day from your intake or burn them through physical activity. Thirty days times 100 calories = 3,000 calories. Multiplied by twelve, this amounts to a loss of 36,000 calories per year—twelve pounds. If you eliminate 200 calories per day from your diet, you will lose two pounds per month for a total of twenty-four in a year. If you eliminate 300, you can drop three pounds in a month, or thirty-six in a year's time.

Conversely, if you *add* to your total caloric intake and do not burn those calories through physical activity, the TCCS equation shows that you will add weight to your body. With the addition of only 100 calories per day, twelve pounds of fat would be added in twelve months, assuming that you don't increase your physical activity to burn off the additional 100 calories ingested. The math looks like this: 100 calories times thirty days times twelve months = 36,000 calories (or twelve pounds) gained per year. For the purposes of this discussion, this is as much detail as I will go into regarding the biochemistry of nutrition. Clearly, other factors also come into play. For example, muscle weighs more than fat. This means that when muscle-building activities are included in one's life plan, weight might be gained or remain the same even as fat is lost. In a future chapter, I'll address the exercise and fitness component of your lifelong weight-management routine.

By now, I hope that you have come to the realization that I identify as a pragmatist. I realize that it is human to stray from the straight and narrow path. Rarely is it possible to adhere to the diet that you know is in your best interest 100 percent of the time. On some days, especially during holidays, we might exceed our required number of calories. For a few days following those special days, we need to (to use the example of a checking account) give back—that is, take away from our calorie-containing intake—the extra calories we ingested during those special occasions. I emphasize the term "calorie counting" above because some foods do not contain calories. For example, the calorie factor for a stalk of celery is minus two calories. On average, it takes two calories of energy to chew and ingest the stalk. The same can be said for other raw leafy vegetables, including iceberg lettuce.

While the following might be more than you want to know about what actually goes on inside your body, the fact is that the only food product that our brains can function with is sugar, and our brains regulate every function of our bodies, both the conscious and subconscious elements. So every food source—carbohydrates, proteins, and fats—must ultimately be broken down into sugars. But we must also keep in mind how—and at what rate—the conversion process takes place.

Another fact to consider in your personalized weight-management plan is that a gram of carbohydrates (simple and complex sugars) contains four calories, each of which produces short-term food value. The reason for the short-lived food value of ingested sugars is that they immediately enter the bloodstream from our stomachs and are quickly converted to energy. On the other hand, a gram of protein contains an equal number of calories (four) but satisfies our hunger urge for a longer period of time.

Conversion of proteins to sugars takes longer and requires more energy than when simple sugars are ingested.

At the other end of the spectrum, a gram of fat contains nine calories and—because it takes longer to convert fat to sugars—satisfies food cravings for an even longer period of time. And the conversion of protein or fat to sugar requires calories. All foods (whether ingested or cannibalized) that contain calories are eventually converted to sugar. Remember, sugar is the only source of energy the human brain can process. And, when all else fails, the brain is created to demand its share of all available resources.

Except for a small amount of complex carbohydrates (sugars) stored in the liver, calories above and beyond those required—regardless of in what form they are ingested—are converted to fat.

If and when a state of starvation occurs, the liver's stored carbohydrates are a body's first source of energy, followed by fat. When all stored fat has been used up, the body begins to break down and converts muscle (protein) to sugar. The process of calling upon reserve sources of energy is known as a catabolic nutritional state, meaning the body is literally feeding upon itself, going through a process that might be called self-cannibalism.

In every *intentional* weight-loss initiative, it is necessary for us, as body owners, to force our bodies into a catabolic (starvation) state. If—and when—the desired amount of weight loss has been achieved, the catabolic state (self-cannibalization) must be arrested. Otherwise, the body will be forced toward a malnourished condition known as anorexia—a state of existence driven by thoughts of negative self-image harbored in the mind, and a state in which psychological intervention is often necessary. If you or someone you know and care about suffers from self-induced anorexia, it means that you or your loved one is unable to let go of the image of a fat version of the self that has been implanted in the mind. This condition has a name—body dysmorphic disorder (BDD). I elaborate on this disorder in a chapter toward the end of this book.

To create a steady state of balance for the patient suffering from BDD requires not only psychological counseling to change the mind's self-image; once the condition is rectified, the exact number of calories expended in a day must be calculated and ingested or exceeded. BDD could be considered an addiction to an altered self-image; therefore, interventional addiction programs are often helpful. Like other matters related to health and appearance that I address in this book, balance is the key—never too much or too little of anything.

During the first several days of any weight-loss program, you might experience a rather rapid reduction in the reading on your scale. This reduction in weight usually results from the loss of fluids that tend to accumulate in your body with the intake of certain foods and spices. It is common knowledge that salt causes the body to retain fluid, but in some individuals, yeast can also lead to fluid retention. Yeast can be found in many baked goods, such as breads, cakes, cookies, and snacks. It is also found in beer, wine, liqueurs, and other fermented alcoholic beverages. In most dieting programs, simple carbohydrates (sugars) and yeast-containing foods and snacks are the first to be eliminated. As a result, diuresis (the release of retained body fluids through the kidneys) occurs. Another phenomenon that is not often associated with weight loss is diarrhea. I call it the diarrhea of dieting. In most cases, it lasts only a few days and is an indication that your body is responding positively to the reduction in calorie intake.

As your intestinal tract is emptied, you will also experience another pound or two of weight loss. It is a normal phenomenon, so do not be alarmed, and do not take measures to stop it—unless, of course, it becomes severe and prolonged. With prolonged bouts of diarrhea, your body will become depleted of potassium, and you will notice that you are becoming weaker. Orange juice and bananas are good sources of potassium replacement.

In an earlier section of this chapter, I mentioned a gift that was given to each of us at the time of our creation: free will. That gift can be both a blessing and a curse, as in the case of morbidly obese individuals when it comes to the will to lose or gain weight. As I stated above, the vast majority of morbidly obese individuals who choose to let their weight get out of control *in the first place* (and choose to take only temporary measures to lose it) generally choose to gain back the weight lost. I say *choose* because—as pointed out earlier—free will gives us the ability to choose how much and what kinds of food and drink we allow to pass through our lips. This confirms an age-old adage: the one who gives the gifts of health, happiness, and prosperity to oneself also possesses the free will to take them away. In that regard, weight management is at least as much an exercise in mental discipline as physical. Overeating and undereating are both examples of addictive behavior, and because they are, that means that they are equally difficult to overcome. We can only arrive at one conclusion: the only long-term solution to weight management is self-discipline—mind over matter. By exercising the gift of free will, we place our minds—not our stomachs—in charge. We give our minds permission to permanently reject old, self-destructive habits and replace them with new, healthy habits. Without exercising this gift, managing one's weight—and remaining healthy—is a lost cause.

A friend once shared an aphorism that applies to becoming comfortable with your new weight-management commitment. The pathway to the brain can be compared to a path through a field. You can walk the old path, or you can choose to create a new path. The old one will always be there, but the more you walk the new one, the more the old, grown-over one will fade in your memory and in the landscape.

The short solution to weight management is to give ourselves a new path—a healthy attitude toward food—and remain disciplined despite the temptations thrown at us. Here are a few other tips to consider:
- Weigh daily.
- Count calories.
- Determine the number of calories needed each day to maintain the desired weight.
- Balance caloric intake with the amount of physical activity expended, just as we would balance our checking or debit account—money deposited versus money spent, calories taken in versus calories expended.

Best results are usually obtained through a healthy combination of physical activity and self-monitored daily caloric intake—for life.

A key to maintaining a given weight often overlooked is to clear our closets of our "fat wardrobe." Give the fat wardrobe away; then resist purchasing larger size clothes. When our "thin" clothes become uncomfortably tight, exercise the discipline to lose back to the point where they fit comfortably, and repeat when necessary.

So, it is rather easy so see that exercising the discipline to adopt—and adhere to—the simple math equation presented in this chapter is the long-lost "secret" to weight management and a better quality of life for you and those who love you. Now that you are beginning to learn how you can take control of your life and become the person of your dreams, you're ready to take a more in-depth look at the nutrition factor.

CHAPTER 9

Smart Nutrition:

Feeding Your Body

Your body is made up of millions of cells. This is a fact that I was taught in high school biology, and I assume that you were as well. Perhaps that's where you learned the following: regardless of its source, we must agree that every cell in your body is in a constant state of change—a state that leads to reproducing itself and then dying off. Depending upon the organ in which a cell is found, the time between its creation, duplication, and demise varies. For example, cells that make up the digestive tract might duplicate themselves every few days. Those that make up the skeletal system (bones and cartilage) replicate only every few months. It stands to reason that the health of the parent cell is crucial to the health of the newly created cell. Simply stated, healthy cells produce healthy cells, and unhealthy cells produce unhealthy cells. And the health of any cell in your body depends upon the nutrients you choose to feed it. In that respect, the gift you give to every cell in your body—and thus to the body of your dreams—is to provide your cells with everything they need in order to do what they were created to do: keep you healthy.

A few years back, my wife was beginning to feel physically and mentally tired by midday. The only way she could get through the remainder of the day was to take a nap. When I became aware of her condition, I suggested that we conduct some tests to see whether she was suffering from a nutritional deficiency. I had already conducted tests that showed that her blood levels of thyroid hormone were lower than optimal and placed her on thyroid supplements. Within days, she began to have more energy and to be more tolerant of cold weather and saw a reduction in the hair loss she had been experiencing over the past several years.

But I did not stop there. I performed micronutrient testing, which measures a person's nutritional health at the cellular level. The tests demonstrated that she had a severe deficiency of one of the body's essential amino acids—a building block for healthy muscle function and regeneration. From my ongoing interest in athletics, I knew that this amino acid deficiency was often seen in distance runners. Susan is not a distance runner; however, the additional testing I performed on her demonstrated that she was deficient in the same essential amino acid, a building block of protein. Upon receiving the results of her test, I prescribed a nutritional supplement program designed to address her deficiency. Within days, she began to feel better. Her midday naps are no longer necessary. Like the Eveready Bunny, she is able to work through the day and turns out original pieces of art more rapidly than most of her fellow artists.

Without micronutrient testing, I might not have been able to diagnose my wife's rare—but real—malnutrition condition, and she might not have been honored in 2017 as "Artist of the Year" by the largest circulated publication within the art world, *ArtTour International*. She might not have received numerous other honors within her profession or served as a trustee of the United States Sports Academy, an institution of higher learning that also contains the world's largest collection of sports art. And our lives together could have been limited.

I continue my discussion of scientific dietary supplementation from the outside-in approach. Your skin is more than a body suit covering the muscles, bones, and systems beneath. As your body's largest biological organ, your skin depends upon proper nutrition, and in order to produce vitamin D, a *reasonable* amount of sunlight is required. Notice that I emphasize the word *reasonable*. Excessive exposure to sunlight can increase your risk of developing skin cancer and seeing the signs of aging creep in at a younger age than genetically programmed.

In order to establish the significance of smart nutrition, I offer the following. If an infant is deprived of essential foods, vitamins, and minerals, the child fails to develop properly. In pediatric circles, the condition is called "failure to thrive." The same condition exists with every infant cell your body produces throughout its lifetime. As discussed above, at every age, each new cell is a baby cell and must be nourished accordingly, or it will fail to thrive and begin to appear unhealthy and older than it should at a stage of your life earlier than normal.

While your skin's external appearance provides clues to the overall state of your health, the only way to know for sure whether the cells and organs beneath are being properly nourished is through scientific testing. Tests that can measure your body's nutritional status have been a long time coming; however, with a sample of your blood, virtually every vitamin, mineral, and amino acid (the building blocks of collagen and elastin production) in your body can now be measured. As in my wife's case, if and when cellular levels of these nutritional elements are found to be deficient in your body's cells, the right combination and amount of the lacking nutrients can be added to your dietary program by a professional consultant. The same is true if the circulating blood levels of essential nutrients are found to be higher than required. You will be instructed to reduce the foods and supplements that are overloading the cells throughout your body.

So many of us take vitamins and supplements on a daily basis yet have no clue as to whether we are taking the right combination or doses. The recommended doses and frequencies listed on the sides of the bottles might not be the dose your body needs. They are simply "recommended" by the company that produces the vitamins. I strongly recommend against taking megadoses of vitamins and supplements without knowing how much, if any, of a given supplement your body actually needs. Periodic retesting will also let you and your health-care professional monitor your nutritional program and adjust it accordingly.

Follow-up monitoring of your supplement program is critical because, if taken in excess, some vitamins can accumulate within the fat cells of your body and might actually be detrimental to your health. Vitamins A, D, E, and K are fat-soluble vitamins. Too much vitamin A can cause symptoms such as liver damage, vision disturbances, nausea, and even death. Vitamin D toxicity can cause a buildup of calcium in your blood (hypercalcemia), which can cause nausea and vomiting, weakness, and frequent urination. Longtime use of large doses of vitamin E over months or years can interfere with your blood's ability to clot in the case of injury or during surgery. Occasionally, muscle weakness, fatigue, nausea, and diarrhea can also occur with excessive intake of vitamin E (fish oil or omega supplements).

Too much vitamin K is rare, but can be detrimental to patients with diabetes in that it can lower blood sugar to levels beyond those intended by prescribed medications. High blood levels of vitamin K can also interfere with medications prescribed by your doctor to prevent your blood from clotting more rapidly than it should, in order to reduce the possibility of stroke and heart attack. It can also interfere with dialysis treatment in patients suffering from kidney failure. So, you can see that every vitamin, supplement, or medication has side effects or might bring risk factors to your health, especially those supplements that are stored in your body. The bottom line is that vitamin and mineral supplements can be dangerous to your health and well-being.

Water-soluble vitamins—that is, every vitamin except A, D, E, and K—do not accumulate in your body. What your body doesn't need will be excreted through your urinary system. Megadose treatments with water-soluble vitamins have often been described by medical skeptics as a way to create expensive urine. As a self-identified pragmatist, when it comes to supplements, I also recommend moderation—not too much or too little—and periodic tests to check your blood levels.

I hope that this overview of vitamins will be sufficient to cause you to take whatever you are putting into your body seriously, for self-treatment can often be dangerous treatment.

Today, there is no need for guesswork—no excuse for risking vitamin toxicity or deficiencies. The cost of learning whether your supplement regimen is providing the cells of your body with the right combinations and doses of nutrients is well worth the dollars and time spent. A growing number of health-insurance plans cover the costs of nutritional testing. I recommend that you check with your provider to see whether your plan does. Even if your company does not cover the cost, micronutrient testing can be performed for about $200 in most areas of the country. If you take vitamins, supplemental minerals, and amino acids, you'll spend that much anyway without knowing whether you are spending your money wisely or risking your health.

Here's another little-known fact about vitamins and supplements. There are different grades, meaning differences in how the products are manufactured. The absorption factor must not be underestimated. Unless a pill can be broken down by your digestive system and each of its ingredients can penetrate the walls of your digestive tract's blood vessels, no supplement can do what is expected. The pill just passes through your digestive system totally or partly intact.

I often use the following example with my patients. You can go out into your yard and pick up a rock—any rock. That rock contains some of the same minerals that are essential for the overall health of your body. However, if you swallow those minerals in the form of a rock retrieved from your yard, they will pass through your digestive system protected by the rock's consistency, and the minerals contained within will be of no use to your body. That's why, as an informed body owner, pharmaceutical-grade vitamins that are manufactured to be fully absorbed into your bloodstream (and thus distributed to every cell within your body) are your best investment.

The first—and least effective—grades of vitamins are those that are required to pass only veterinary standards and are not subject to the multilevel scrutiny of the US Food and Drug Administration. Veterinary-grade vitamins and supplements can be obtained through mail-order catalogues at a fraction of the cost of the more effective grades. In humans, the absorbability of this grade of vitamins is suspect at best. Therefore, their effectiveness remains questionable.

The second grade of vitamins and supplements are those that are available in drug and grocery stores. In most cases, the absorbability of these supplements is better than the veterinary grade but falls short of the higher grades.

The third grade comprises those supplements sold by health-supplement chains or so-called "health-food stores," usually located in shopping centers. They tend to be a bit more absorbable—and thus more effective—but still fall short of the gold standard of dietary supplementation, pharmaceutical-grade supplements.

Pharmaceutical-grade supplements are usually provided by physicians or physician extenders. In a nutshell, the difference in the grades addressed above in is the product's ability to find their way into your body's bloodstream. It is the only way that micronutrients can be put to their intended use throughout your body, except—in rare cases—by intravenous administration.

I cannot overstate that without conducting laboratory tests that scientifically measure your blood's existing levels of the necessary building blocks of smart and healthy nutrition, there is no way to know whether you need nutritional supplements or whether the most appropriate combinations or dosages are being administered to you. Furthermore, because over-the-counter vitamins and supplements are classified by the US Food and Drug Administration as "foods," they are not subject to the regulations required of physician-prescribed products.

The takeaway message of this chapter is that if you are inclined to supplement your diet with vitamins and minerals, make sure you know what—if any—nutritional elements are actually deficient within your body. Any remedy you undertake (self-administered or otherwise) should be monitored or overseen by a trained health-care professional who is both capable of and willing to conduct periodic testing in order to monitor the nutritional health of every cell within your body—the body of your dreams.

The next section addresses another arena of bodily supplementation, one that—because you are a human being—will ultimately be required in order to maintain your well-being, appearance, performance, and productivity.

CHAPTER 10

The Effects of Hormones and Stress on Aging

There is no debate among health-care professionals that hormone levels drop with every year past the age of thirty. In women, the process happens rapidly, causing obvious changes in the way a woman feels and looks—an often dreaded process known as menopause. In men, the process is known as andropause and occurs more gradually, often sparing males of flash sweats, mood swings, and fluid retention. However, by the age of fifty, both men and women experience measurable drops in essential hormones that were once produced by the endocrine system. Optimal levels of those hormones help us sustain a youthful appearance, heightened performance, and a positive outlook on life.

The bad news is that optimal levels of hormones steadily decrease as we age. The good news is that, in the hands of a mind/body/spirit specialist, deficient hormone levels can be replaced with biocompatible compounds. I prefer the term *compatible* because unless the product is derived from human sources, it is not *identical*.

A common medication long prescribed to offset the signs and symptoms of menopause is a supplement known as Premarin—phonetically *pre-mar-in*. These three syllables are derived from the words "pregnant mares' urine." That this estrogen-replacement product is derived from horse hormones means that it might not be as effective as products derived from other sources, such as yams. I recommend that you ask your doctor about the sources of biocompatible hormone-replacement products that might be available to you.

Although I am primarily a surgeon, before the facial plastic surgery and Rejuvenology years of my training, I served an externship with UAB's OB-GYN department and personally delivered scores of babies over a period of two months. At the time, more babies were delivered at UAB than at any other hospital in the Birmingham, Alabama, area. As part of my duties, I also provided pre- and postnatal care at UAB's OB-GYN clinics.

Upon completion of those duties, I returned to the medical/surgical curriculum required of UAB medical students. In addition, however, I took an after-hours job as an autopsy prosector with UAB's Department of Pathology. Then, while a resident in otolaryngology and head and neck surgery and as a fellow in facial plastic surgery, I also served as the first official medical director of nursing homes in the state of Alabama. Before I created the position within the Estes nursing home corporation, nursing homes did not have medical directors. They only had doctors who took care of the patients' health conditions. During a five-year period, I did both. I developed protocols for education, treatment, and management for the patients and staff of each facility. I also provided care and counsel to thousands of senior citizens who were confined to nursing home care.

Collectively, each of the experiences addressed above gave me a cradle-to-grave insight into the cycle of life that few physicians experience. As a medical director and physician for hundreds of nursing home patients, I experienced the physical, psychological, financial, and social aspects of the birthing and aging processes and everything in between.

While some readers might view the insight and recommendations I offer as philosophical in nature, my views are based upon a solid foundation—a lifetime devoted to studying the creation and divinely engineered evolution of the human species. My studies are garnished with a healthy dose of my personal experiences as a caregiver solemnly sworn to the Hippocratic oath. I consider it a responsibility to share as many of those experiences with you as possible in this venue.

The Stress Factor: How to Speed Up or Slow Down the Aging Process

With each passing year, research scientists are learning more about the aging process. I view this as an example of what I refer to in *Let Us Make Man* as divinely engineered creative evolution—a brilliantly engineered process through which a being created in the image of God and His angels is also allowed to participate in its own evolutionary journey. While no one has yet discovered how to arrest the aging process and remain alive, it is well documented how the aging process can be accelerated.

As numerous prophetic writers have chronicled—and as I can affirm—the secret to slowing down the aging process is a gift originally given to each, and every, body owner by our Creator(s)—a gift that resides within the mind and spirit of each and every one of us. I have labeled that gift self-care. One way to exercise self-care is to find ways to reduce the stress in our lives that causes us to age more quickly than we might otherwise experience.

While we might have all been created from a common set of parents (the metaphorical Adam and Eve), one fact remains: with the exception of those of us with handicaps, the rest of us are duly equipped to function within the environments in which we were born. Even though we share a common heritage, each of us tends to respond to the same circumstances in somewhat different ways as a result of mind-sets created, in part, from previous life experiences and the manner in which we chose to deal with them.

As both Dr. Samuel Smiles and Dr. Orison Marden have pointed out (and as mind/body aficionado James Allen has echoed), it is how each of us responds to the challenges we face that determines the effects those conditions have upon our minds and bodies. Clearly, some people absorb and harbor stress like a sponge takes on water. Others shed stress like Teflon resists the same external forces. Because they drown in their own misery, the sponge segment of our species is more apt to experience the physical and mental effects of stress than our Teflon counterparts. The Teflon segment chooses to view every roadblock as a detour—an alternate way to a strategically charted destination.

Dr. Marden tells a story about a young woman who, after her lover jilted her on their supposed wedding day, was committed to an insane asylum. Perhaps you are familiar with this saying: "The insane have solved their problems. They simply retreated from the reality their minds chose to suppress in order to protect the host from doom and gloom." Because this woman's mind was frozen in time, in her seventies she exhibited none of the typical signs associated with aging. She did not have wrinkles or gray hair. In her self-protective Teflon mind, time stood still, and the factors that would have caused her to age never weighed heavily on her.

The sponge segment of our species would view the same set of circumstances as a load too heavy to carry and allow it to break their backs (metaphorically) or spirits. This rather simplistic example of stress management might be as valid an explanation for the stress-ending alternative known as suicide. I remind readers that the term could apply to the physical, mental, or vocational state of being. Yet stress might be one of the most correctable enemies of longevity, productivity, and happiness. It is not the fact that stress exists in our lives that determines its effect on us; it is how we choose to deal with stress.

Whether dementia is related to a body owner's mind's attempt to protect itself from the dreaded physical and emotional aspects of aging is a thought that should be explored. Clearly the jilted bride's mind shut down some of its thought processes in order to protect her from dealing with a painful reality. What is the possibility that dementia might be related—in part—to the same process? Just a thought.

Professionally overseen stress relief might be one of the most effective ways to arrest the unwanted signs and symptoms of aging and ensure prolonged mental health. A period of aerobic exercise, relaxation, or meditation is also effective in releasing pent-up stress. A professionally administered therapeutic facial or body massage relaxes the muscles and mind. Both are examples of the age-honored healing method known as the "laying on of hands" by an individual believed—in the mind of the recipient—to be a caregiver. In addition to providing the placebo effect, both lower tension levels and create the release of the body's own natural chemical relaxants and painkillers (endorphins.) This—coupled with reflexology therapy and the peaceful, professional environment that exists in most spas—allow our minds to let go of the kinds of pent-up tension that promote premature aging. At the same time, the ability to handle tension and thus offset premature aging increases productivity in the workplace and helps create happier environments in our home settings.

Keep in mind that there are different kinds of massages. Some tend to release more of your body's endorphins than others. Ask your therapist which is best for stress relief. The kind of massage that works for a friend or family member might not be the best choice for you. Yoga and related disciplines, along with massage therapy, might also lessen the amount of painkillers you need and thus reduce the risk of becoming dependent on such medications. Keep in mind that self-medication can be a danger to your overall health and well-being.

Like many of the remedies I address in this book, yoga gets a body owner in touch with the body's physical, mental, and spiritual components. This gives yoga high marks as a way for you to relax, manage your stress and anxiety, and achieve peacefulness in your body and mind at the times you most need it.

When the pressures of stress or the weight of lingering grief becomes too heavy to manage, I recommend that you seek the services of a licensed counselor or therapist who possesses the training and experience to assist you through such times. You must not view asking for help under these circumstances as a sign of weakness. Seeking the assistance of a trained professional is a demonstration of wisdom—one of the gifts you give yourself on the way to becoming the person of your dreams.

CHAPTER 11

Enhancement Medicine and Surgery

After an excursion through the nonsurgical appearance enhancement-industry, we now return to the most reliable and time-tested methods of helping you become the person of your dreams. Even among some branches of the medical profession, confusion exists when it comes to many of the terms used to describe life-enhancement medicine and surgery. Because we are about to embark on that aspect of your self-giving journey, I thought a glossary would be helpful as we move toward the more medical and surgical options available to people like you who are focused on becoming the best you that you can be.

I encourage you to read the chapters that follow. While you might currently be one of those individuals who say, "I'll never have plastic surgery," the fact that you know about these options will make you a more informed consumer. And keep in mind that a closed mind is a mind that knows not how to dream great dreams.

These are some of the terms that you will hear discussed in circles where people freely talk about becoming the person of their dreams.

- **Abdominoplasty:** Tummy tuck; removal of excess skin and fat of the lower abdomen, often coupled with tightening of stretched abdominal muscles.
- **Aesthetic Surgery:** Appearance-enhancement surgery; another term for cosmetic surgery.
- **Blepharoplasty:** Surgical removal of excess fat or skin from the upper or lower eyelids.
- **Board-Certified Surgeon:** One who has completed an accredited residency (or specialty) training program and who has passed a comprehensive examination in their field of study.
- **Chemabrasion:** A chemical peel; the use of selective chemicals on the face that cause the top layers of skin to peel away, producing

smoother, more youthful skin that is less likely to form cancerous changes.

- **Cosmetic Plastic Surgery:** Another term for aesthetic plastic surgery; procedures designed to enhance one's appearance.
- **Dermabrasion:** Surgical buffing of the top layers of skin to improve or remove facial wrinkles or irregularities caused by scarring from acne or injury.
- **Eyelid Tuck**: A procedure performed at some point following a blepharoplasty in order to provide tightening of newly formed eyelid skin and fat pads.
- **Facial Plastic Surgeon:** A surgeon who specializes in plastic and reconstructive surgery of the face, nose, head, and neck.
- **Facial Tuck:** A procedure performed at some point following a facelift in order to provide tightening of new facial tissues that formed as a result of a continuation of the aging process.
- **Hair Restoration:** Use of plasma rich protein (PRP) on areas of the scalp where hair is beginning to thin.
- **Hair Transplantation:** Surgical transfer of hair-bearing grafts to areas of baldness.
- **Hypertrophic Scar:** A thick, wide, and sometimes painful scar.
- **Integrative Medicine:** "An approach to care that puts the patient at the center and addresses the full range of physical, emotional, mental, social, spiritual and environmental influences that affect a person's health. . . . It uses the most appropriate interventions from an array of scientific disciplines to heal illness and disease and help people regain and maintain optimum health."[6]
- **Keloid:** An enlarged scar that extends beyond the boundaries of the original injury or incision site.
- **Laser Surgery:** The use of an intensified beam of light to vaporize tissue.

---

6. "What Is Integrative Medicine?," Duke Integrative Medicine, accessed September 30, 2019, https://dukeintegrativemedicine.org/about/what-is-integrative-medicine/.

- **Mammaplasty:** Surgical alteration of the size and shape of breasts, including augmentation (enlarging the breasts by the insertion of medical-grade implants) or reduction (reducing the size of the breast by removing excess tissues).
- **Mastopexy:** The breast-lift operation.
- **Mentoplasty:** Otherwise known as chin augmentation, this procedure involves building up the chin, often using an implant or a repositioning of the patient's own bone and soft tissues.
- **Microdermabrasion:** Superficial exfoliation of the very top layer of skin to provide temporary improvement in the skin's texture.
- **Otoplasty:** The reshaping and repositioning of protruding or deformed ears.
- **Plastic Surgeon:** A specialist who practices plastic and reconstructive surgery of the entire body (face, breast, abdomen, extremities, etc.).
- **Plastic Surgery:** A field of surgery comprised of both cosmetic (aesthetic) and reconstructive procedures designed to enhance, restore, or reconstruct body parts.
- **Reconstructive Plastic Surgery:** Procedures designed to restore the body to a normal state.
- **Rejuvenology:** The combined arts and sciences devoted to appearance and health enhancement.
- **Rhinoplasty:** A procedure used to alter the width, size, or shape of the nose. Often combined with a septoplasty to improve breathing and relieve headaches.
- **Rhytidectomy:** The facelift operation; a surgical procedure that removes excess skin, following the suspension of sagging muscles and connective tissue in the face and neck.
- **Scalp Flaps:** A repositioning of large portions of hair-bearing scalp onto areas of baldness.
- **Suction Lipectomy:** Liposuction; the vacuuming or suctioning of unwanted fat using cannulae inserted beneath the skin.

Getting to Truth

Although it might not be clear which comes first—beauty, health, happiness, or prosperity—they are, no doubt, symbiotic, meaning they feed upon and enhance each other. And it doesn't really matter at which age you choose to be all that you can be. Providing you faithfully follow the recommendations and admonitions offered within this book, the results should be measurable and long lasting and should pay big dividends.

To provide a broad understanding of facial rejuvenation surgery, I developed the following classification. It addresses the various stages of aging and the surgical procedures that are available to stabilize or reverse them. Because biological ages do not always match chronological ages, some individuals within the same age group will exhibit more—or less—aging than their peers. A number of factors contribute to this, including genetics, lifestyle, stress, nutrition, nicotine, and excessive alcohol use.

Surgery that addresses facial aging must focus on more than sagging skin of the cheeks and neck. The truth is that while a "facelift" might be part of the plan, if the best results are to be obtained, more than traditional face lifting should be considered. Many patients will benefit from work on drooping eyebrows or upper and lower eyelids to remove bags and sags in those regions. Individuals with wrinkles, acne scars, and sun-damaged skin might want to consider one of the skin-resurfacing procedures mentioned in chapter 22. For the best results, some patients require liposuction in the lower cheeks and neck. In fact, patients under the age of forty might require nothing more than facial and neck liposuction, after which their elastic, youthful skin will contract to conform to the newly sculpted shape of the face and neck.

It is important to recognize that a number of accessorizing procedures can also be carried out at the same time as face lifting without adding to recovery times, including procedures performed on the nose, eyelids, lips, body, arms, hands, and legs.

A fundamental principle within medical circles is that diagnosis precedes treatment. A corollary to this principle is that the *right* diagnosis combined with the *right* treatment is apt to yield better outcomes. Based on these irrefutable principles, you can only deduce that in order to maintain or recapture a youthful appearance, not all faces and bodies should be subjected to the same procedures. Instead, a long-term and comprehensive rejuvenation plan should be considered prior to the initiation of any treatment, including procedures that can provide only short-term benefits. Your rejuvenation plan ought to be personalized and tailored to meet your needs and desires at every stage of your life.

Keep in mind that not every enhancement professional is capable of providing everything that might be included in your master enhancement and rejuvenation plan. However, a Rejuvenologist who understands the various procedures and products that might come into play should become the coordinator and monitor. Finding this individual might require research and visits to a number of offices before you identify the professional best qualified to serve as the master enhancement planner and overseer.

Unfortunately, you and I live in a society with an unhealthy appetite for short-term goals and instant gratification. Many of these short-lived practices have found their way into the appearance-enhancement industry. The result is that commercialization, not verifiable science, is driving public demand.

In response, many doctors appear to be playing the role of follower rather than leader. For fear of losing patients to other doctors, a growing—yet inadvisable—trend is to give patients what they ask for rather than what is in their best interest. Regrettably, I hear my fellow appearance-enhancing surgeons make such statements before large audiences of colleagues more often than you might imagine. I cannot agree with or condone this approach to patient care. I believe it is our job as physicians and surgeons to recommend the *right* procedures and products at the *right* time in our patients' lives. Only once those recommendations have been made has the doctor fulfilled their responsibility to provide informed consent, a legal term for making sure that a patient understands the treatment that they are about to undergo. Today, patients are asking for procedures and products that television and print commercials encourage them to ask for, many of which are not in their best interests.

Changes within the medical profession itself are also contributing to the dilemma. With the apparent avalanche of government-controlled health care, many doctors whose training consisted of nonsurgical modalities are abandoning medically focused practices and turning to cosmetic procedures as a way to shore up declining incomes.

Technology companies recognize these changes, as well as others taking place throughout the health-care industry. As a result, they are reaching out to doctors from a wide variety of nonsurgical specialties, encouraging them to include laser treatments, injectable therapies, and assembly-line surgical procedures that can be commercially franchised. The danger in such a trend is obvious. Corporate executives, not physicians, end up dictating policy and setting standards.

In recent years, many of the commercialized cosmetic surgery franchises have gone by the wayside. On a massive scale, it is difficult to maintain the degree of quality control to which board-certified surgeons are held. So, here's my recommendation. Before you agree to undergo a commercial-sounding cosmetic procedure, do the research. Ask the hard questions, and do not take generalized answers as the facts. Ask to see pre- and postoperative results that were performed by the surgeon under consideration. Photographs provided by a marketing company or the manufacturer of a device might not be representative of the results obtained by the doctor sitting before you.

The Ideal Enhancement Team

The ongoing process of enhancing and maintaining the shape of your figure or physique requires a cooperative effort that involves your participation and commitment as well as a team of life-enhancement professionals.

When such a plan includes the recommendations I've presented, individuals of all ages and from all walks of life are more likely to match a youthful, attractive face or nose with an equally balanced body, inside and out. When right-minded thought is included in the enhancement process, patients and clients can also rid themselves of unwanted fat, build muscle, and improve the shape and proportions of anatomical regions and features that are either smaller or larger than desired.

Over the past four decades, I have witnessed that individuals who suffer from diabetes, high blood pressure, high cholesterol, arthritis, depression, and many other conditions often see the aforementioned health conditions disappear simply by obtaining—and maintaining—a healthier-looking body.

As with facial surgery, breast and body sculpting procedures, hormonal balancing, dietary and nutritional supplement plans also vary from individual to individual and from medical facility to medical facility. The bottom line is that every body owner must do the research. Ask the hard questions. Insist that the names, specialties, certifications, and licenses of all potential providers are presented willingly and completely. I remind you of a truth that must remain at the forefront of your mind: it is your body, and you have the right to know what is going to be done and who is going to do it. Being your own advocate in the life-enhancement arena is another one of those gifts that you give yourself.

Tilting the Scales of Opportunity

Now that we've looked at the big picture, I'm going to share some real-life examples in which the recommendations and admonitions I offered became more than theory.

The before and after photographs below demonstrate the result of surgery designed to enhance the nose and chin of a young professional woman who needed a boost in her self-esteem.

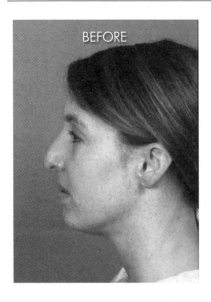 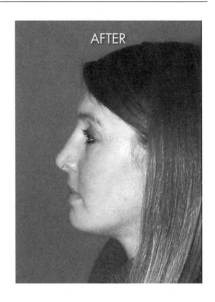

Several months after her surgery, she sent the following letter to me.

Dear Dr. McCollough,

I didn't realize how the surgery you performed would change my life so positively. I find with all the compliments I've received, I've started holding my head up more and making more eye contact with others. I believe this gives me more confidence and the appearance of having more confidence. In turn, I have been entrusted with more meaningful work projects and had more opportunities for success in my career.

I can never thank you enough. I will always remember the kindness of you and your staff, which made my experience with this surgery so delightful.

My response is this: "Thank *you* for allowing me to be your doctor and surgeon. That you would trust me with your appearance and well-being is as great an honor as any caregiver can ask." Almost daily, I hear similar comments from my patients. That's what keeps me coming to work. The opportunity to share these stories with you, the reader, is a privilege I do not take lightly.

CHAPTER 12

Nose-Enhancing Surgery:

The Rhinoplasty Operation

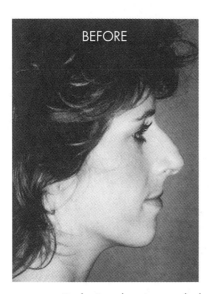 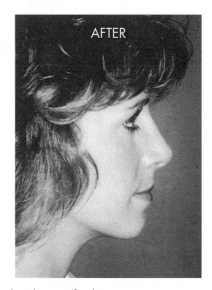

Reducing the size and altering the shape of a large nose
brings it into harmony with other facial features.

Down through history, the human nose has been a subject of attention—
sometimes ridiculed, at other times exploited.

In the case of Cyrano de Bergerac, although he was talented, witty,
and good in a fight, the enormous size of his nose made it impossible,
in his mind, for him to garner the courage to win over female admirers.
Even so, because of who he was on the inside, Cyrano won over the love
of life, Roxanne . . . as he, tragically, died.

In contrast, twentieth-century entertainer Jimmy Durante exploited the size of his larger-than-average nose (which he loving called his
"schnoz") as a way to make him stand out from competing entertainers.
It worked.

However, as it was for the real and mythically embellished Cyrano, most people who have large noses consider them impairments to the realization of their dreams. If they do, it is only after surgical correction that the psychological impairment disappears.

In this chapter, we go beyond myth and examine the facts.

Your nose is the most prominent feature on your face. Like other features, it changes throughout your life. As a child, you likely had a cute pug nose. When you became an adolescent, you developed a bridge, and your nose took on its adult shape. As you age, the nose will change again. The tip will begin to droop, making the hump—assuming you had one—appear larger. If, in your youth, you never had a hump on your nose, you are likely to develop one in your sixties and seventies. So what can you do to change the appearance of your nose and prevent the tip from drooping as you age?

Rhinoplasty is the name of the operation designed to enhance the appearance and function of the nose. In many cases, the nasal airway and sinus health are improved. An often overlooked advantage of rhinoplasty is that patients who have suffered with headaches often find that their headaches disappear or become less frequent and less severe following surgery.

At the end of this chapter, I share another letter received from a patient upon whom I performed a rhinoplasty and, at the same time, corrected a deviated septum (crooked bones and cartilages inside her nose). She shares how this not only improved her self-esteem but eliminated a longstanding history of headaches.

Like faces, every nose is different; some noses are too long, some too wide, some have large humps, some project away from the face, and so on. A skilled rhinoplasty surgeon can assess the conditions inside and outside your nose and recommend the necessary changes.

Because rhinoplasty surgery is as much artistic in nature as it is scientific, rarely are any two patients' noses identical after surgery. The exception is when the procedure is performed on identical twins. In those cases—because the two faces are identical—I attempt to make each twin's nose match the other's.

As much as any appearance-enhancing procedure, rhinoplasty is one that is truly tailored to the patient's individual circumstances. The alterations recommended should be determined by many factors, including the patient's gender, height, age, skin thickness, and ethnic background and the configuration of their other features, such as the forehead, eyes, and chin. All in all, elite rhinoplastic surgeons strive to achieve a natural-looking nose rather than one that appears to have been operated upon. No patient really wants an assembly-line "nose job"; they want a nose individually tailored to their own features and character.

During the procedure, the nose is reduced in size by removing excess bone and cartilage. The remaining structures are reshaped and repositioned through a series of carefully planned internal nasal incisions. In revision or corrective rhinoplasty, it might be necessary to use grafts to replace structural components that were removed by previous surgeries. After the architectural components of the nose are created, the skin then provides a covering over the newly constructed framework.

Are There Age Limits for Rhinoplasty?

People often ask: At what age can nasal plastic and reconstructive surgery be performed? If a severe breathing problem (or headache issue) is present, it should be corrected conservatively, even in a child. And I emphasize *conservatively*. With children, additional surgery at maturity might be required to obtain the optimal result. Certain limitations exist in children that preclude performing the definitive correction prior to puberty; however, by correcting most of the condition, a poor self-image and altered facial development may be avoided.

Ordinarily, girls are mature enough by the age of fifteen (and boys by eighteen) to have surgical correction; however, because some boys and girls mature at earlier ages, it is necessary to individualize this criterion. So that growth and maturation can be monitored, I recommend a consultation for these young men and women whenever they become interested in having a rhinoplasty even if surgical correction will be delayed.

Early correction of unwanted nasal deformities can often give young people more self-confidence and enhance their self-esteem. A parent should come with a minor to the consultation visit.

On the other hand, about 30 percent of the five-thousand-plus rhinoplasties I have performed were on patients over the age of forty. Many patients remark that they have disliked their noses all their life and have now decided to have corrective surgery. Providing you're in good health, it is never too late in life to give yourself a rhinoplasty. It is often performed as a part of a facial rejuvenation program with face lifting and eyelid plastic surgery to improve the signs of aging.

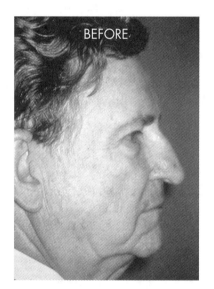 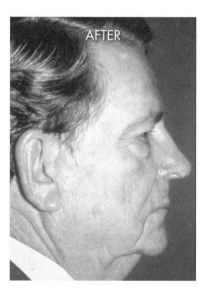

A longer, drooping nose can be a telltale sign of aging.
Repositioning the drooping tip of the nose can give a more
youthful appearance and an improved airway.

The Planning Process

As with all facial surgical procedures, photographs are taken prior to the rhinoplasty so that I can study the characteristics interrelated with the nose within my prospective patient's face. The operation is planned in much the same way an architect plans a house or building. My goal is not only to improve the shape of the nose but also to have it enhance the appearance of the other features of my patient's face.

Medical photographs are helpful in helping me determine whether surgery might be indicated. In many cases, a teleconferenced photographic analysis and interview are conducted prior to an in-office consultation, thereby shortening the time from the first call to operation.

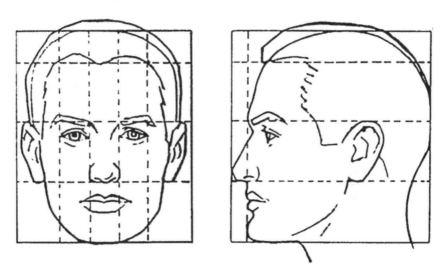

The "ideal" facial proportions are demonstrated in this photograph. The nose should fit into the middle third of the face, as depicted in this diagram. From a profile view, the chin should be in line with the lower lip.

Then there is the following letter, received from a twin who had suffered from debilitating headaches for much of her life. Yet no medical provider had considered a correctable problem inside her nose as the cause of her headaches.

> *Dear Dr. McCollough,*
>
> *It has been seven months since my rhinoplasty and I have never felt better. I am now able to breathe fully through both nostrils for the first time in 30 years. In addition to my better-looking nose, I no longer am troubled with the headaches that I previously experienced almost on a daily basis.*
>
> *I am now living life to the fullest and finally feel like a normal person. My life has been changed forever.*
>
> *K.T.*

Clearly, correcting the appearance and functional aspects of an unhappy nose can change a person's life. That is why, within the appearance- and health-enhancing industries, rhinoplasty is often referred to as the queen of plastic and reconstructive surgery.

The following chapter pertains to the second most defining portion of the face that we inherit from our ancestors: our chin. As you transition from this chapter to the next, you might recall that in an earlier section of this book, I stated that 40 percent of Americans are dissatisfied with the size and shape of their noses and that 25 percent are dissatisfied with their chins.

CHAPTER 13

Chin Enhancement

A few years back, the patient whose photographs are included below consulted with me regarding concerns she had about the appearance of her chin and neck. "It is a family trait," she said, "and continues to worsen with age. Now I'm seeing it happen to me."

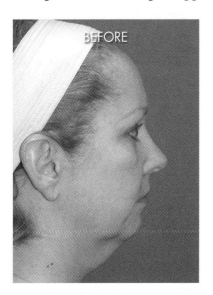
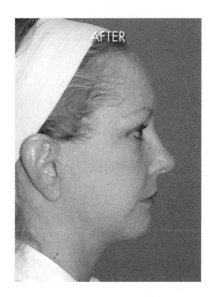

Within families like hers, especially in the members that have smaller chin bones, fat also tends to accumulate in the neck below. As the skin in that region ages, it, too, starts to sag, adding to the underlying structural concerns.

In younger patients, a chin implant (augmentation mentoplasty) alone can correct the deficiency and provide facial harmony. However, if excess fat is already present in the neck below, liposuction is also recommended. Based upon my experience, it does matter which form of liposuction is used. The newly hyped laser-assisted liposuction is no more effective than the standard form that has been used with great success for more than thirty years; nor are so-called nonsurgical injectable products that are designed to dissolve fat.

For the patient whose photographs are included above—and for others in her same age group—a cheek-neck facelift was necessary. Sagging muscles had to be suspended; then the excess skin of her neck was removed.

In keeping with my attempts to provide understanding regarding sometimes complex medical terms, I offer the following. The Greek word for chin is *mentum*. The suffix *-plasty* means "to shape" (referring to shaping some body part). Thus, the medical term for chin enhancement is *mentoplasty*. When the chin is too small for the face, augmentation (adding to it) can often produce dramatic improvement in facial features.

Very often—as was the case in the patient whose photographs I include above—it is necessary to recommend surgery for a receding chin, either in connection with a facelift, liposuction of the neck, or a nasal plastic operation or as an isolated procedure. The reason is that an experienced facial plastic surgeon does not consider the chin to be an isolated structure but rather—as our body-proportion mentor Leonardo da Vinci pointed out—an important feature of the face. More specifically, my appearance-enhancing colleagues and I think in terms of balance and achieving the most aesthetically pleasing profile obtainable for our patients.

Chin augmentation carries a high success rate and, in most cases, adds the finishing touch when reconstructing facial harmony.

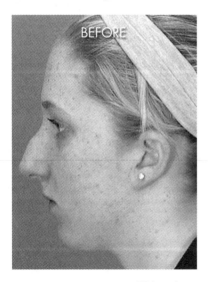 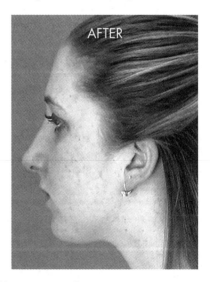

Rhinoplasty and chin augmentation.

Facial Analysis

During a consultation with an appearance-enhancing surgeon, the prospective patient's chin is analyzed to determine whether augmentation should be considered. Generally speaking, if you examine your profile (side view) in a mirror, the ideal chin projection should coincide with a vertical line extending downward from your lower lip.

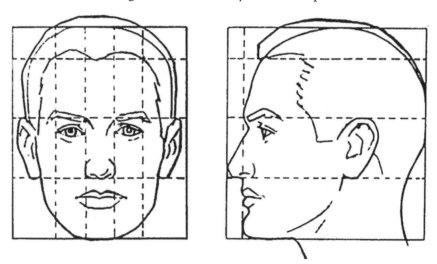

From the profile, the chin alignment should approximate
a line extended vertically from the lower lip.

Too much recession of the chin, particularly when accompanied by a backward-slanting forehead, will cause the features of the face to taper to a point in the midface, especially if only nasal plastic surgery (rhinoplasty) is performed. Actually, we appearance-enhancing surgeons may advise against rhinoplasty unless our patients agree to have the projection of their chin brought into harmony at the same time.

Of course, some people desire chin augmentation alone. In addition to familial predispositions, a receding chin can result from long-term nasal blockage, enlarged adenoids, or dental problems. In such cases, the chin did not develop properly. This is a fact that should be shared with pediatricians and family physicians who treat children.

In my own practice, I prefer to perform chin augmentation through an incision made inside the mouth, just above the crease between the lower lip and the gums. Absorbable sutures are used, and when the scar inside matures, it is not only thread thin but out of sight.

When chin augmentation is performed in conjunction with another procedure, it is not necessary for the patient to recover for any longer than if the other procedure were performed alone. Most patients can resume their preoperative activities within about one week, when the external tapes (which are the skin tone of light-skinned patients) are removed.

For more than four decades, medical-grade mesh has been my implant of choice. The reason is that there is absolutely no evidence that mesh materials dissolve the underlying bone of the patient's chin. The same cannot be said for solid, silicone implant materials.

Chin augmentation is the same concept as one of the most popular cosmetic operations in the world—breast augmentation (mammaplasty). In both procedures, an implant is placed underneath the tissues of the body it is intended to enhance. In the chin operation, the implant is placed directly on top of the patient's jawbone so that the soft tissues (skin, fat, and muscles) come to rest upon the implant rather than upon the bone itself.

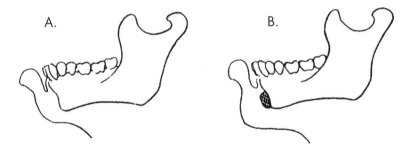

(a) A receding chin is usually the result of a short mandible (jaw bone). An implant (b) placed on the mandible supports the tissues, bringing the chin into better alignment.

Medical-grade mesh-like materials are not new. Regardless of some of the negative press they have received in recent years, mesh implants are also employed to make artificial heart components and arteries. They are also used for reconstruction around the eye and nose, for repairing hernias, and for many other purposes in various parts of the body. These materials have been used in many cases and enjoy a high record of safety and satisfaction; however, as can occur with any implantable material, infection is always a possibility. Among the many advantages of using mesh implants is that after a short time has elapsed, the patient's own tissues fill in the spaces between the mesh. Therefore, the implant serves as a matrix, becoming practically the same consistency as the surrounding tissues and incorporating into them.

The next chapter deals with structures closely related to the chin: lips. You are likely to be introduced to facts about lip enhancement to which you have not previously been exposed.

CHAPTER 14

Lip Enhancement:

Lifting and Augmentation

Since the turn of the twenty-first century, more and more people have become interested in having youthful, full lips.

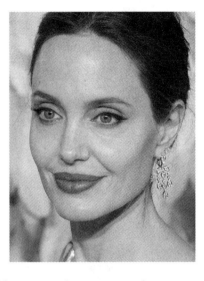

This fact affirms another point I wish to make. Celebrities tend to drive the definitions of beauty and handsomeness. Angelina Jolie comes to mind. The size of her full lips— among her other naturally appealing attributes—created a movement in the appearance-enhancement world.

As previously mentioned, injectable materials can provide temporary enhancement to your lips; however, as a facial plastic surgeon with decades of experience, I have seen temporary solutions to appearance enhancement vault onto the scene and then disappear almost as rapidly. Based on those years of experience, I tend to recommend enhancement procedures and products that provide long-term improvement. Although surgical correction might not be recommended for every face, a surgical lip lift or an anatomical graft using a strip of the patient's own collagen can offer a more permanent improvement to individuals concerned about congenitally thin or aging lips. When the cost of repeated injections is taken into consideration, surgical correction can prove to be the more economical route to pursue.

I recall the case of a woman who traveled to see me from Washington, DC. She was there to consult with me about enlarging her ever-thinning lips. During our consultation, she admitted to having poor self-esteem and resisted having preoperative photographs taken, even though they were to be taken in a controlled medical setting.

The following day, I performed a lip advancement and augmentation procedure using carefully harvested strips of her own collagen, obtained from the creases behind her ears. She returned several months later for a follow-up visit. Her before and after photographs are included below.

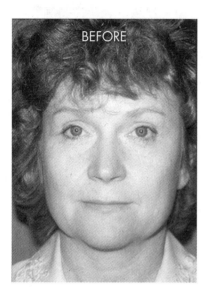
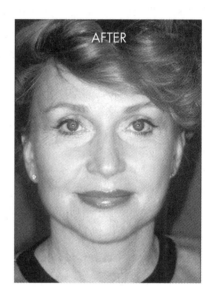

On her return visit, she told me that she had read in a Washington, DC, newspaper that a James Bond movie was going to be filmed in the area and that the producers were looking for extras for the opening scene—a wedding party that was to take place around a backyard swimming pool. She had auditioned for the part and had been hired. The patient who had, a few months before, resisted having her photographs taken in a controlled medical environment had come to feel so confident that she was willing to audition against hundreds of candidates and have her image captured by multiple movie cameras. As you study the photographs above, I also draw your attention to the fact that this patient also began to use makeup, style her hair, wear accessorizing items, and upgrade her wardrobe.

Hers is a story that I have witnessed hundreds of times throughout my career. Features that others might advise against having enhanced are often viewed by those who possess those features as psychological albatrosses around their necks. This patient gave herself the opportunity to address the features that—in her mind—negatively affected her self-esteem and confidence. That she chose to undergo appearance-enhancing surgery meant that she gave herself the ability to become the person of her dreams. That she competed for—and landed—a role in a James Bond movie is a testament to the self-confidence she gained from a simple procedure that took less than an hour to perform.

As I share this patient's story, I am reminded of a statement often quoted by one of my own mentors, Dr. Jack R. Anderson: "A person who is suffering with a feature that affects their self-image can either lie on a therapist's couch for two years and learn to live with the feature or lie down on an operating room table for two hours or less and have that feature corrected."

Whereas in the previous chapter on chin augmentation I recommend an implant (something that is not part of a patient's body) as the best solution for enhancing a receding or small chin, I adamantly recommend against artificial implants in the lips. If augmentation (by filling) is to be performed, I prefer to use a strip of my patient's own collagen, which can be obtained from behind the ears or, in conjunction with a facelift, from in front of the patient's ears.

With aging, the fullness of everyone's lips begins to subside—sometimes to the extent that most of the thin pink membrane disappears from view. In these cases, something other than collagen grafts is required. The junction line between the skin of the lips needs to be advanced outward and upward in the upper lip and outward and downward in the lower lip. This procedure is known as a lip lift.

In patients with white skin, the procedure is performed by removing a strip of the white skin around the lip and advancing the pink skin into the defect. Tiny incisions are made in the corners of the mouth and underneath the lip in the center. With a couple of weeks, the incision sites are invisible.

For white-skinned patients beyond the age of forty, lip-enhancement surgery is often combined with a skin-resurfacing procedure (chemical peel, dermabrasion, or laser), especially when wrinkles are present.

I have never seen a patient with black skin request to have their lips enlarged. On the contrary, patients whose ancestors, ancient or recent, originated in Africa often wish to have their lips reduced in size. In order to achieve this objective, tissue is removed from inside the lip. Because the incisions are made inside their lips—rather than in the skin of their faces—the resulting scars are imperceptible.

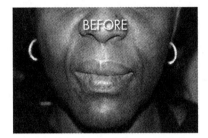 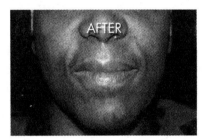

In my decades of enhancing the noses, faces, lips, and lives of patients from all walks of life, I have never seen a keloid—often dreaded—develop on the membranes of the lips and mouth, nor am I familiar with any such report in the annals of plastic and reconstructive surgery.

Since 1998, I have been enhancing the lips of younger white-skinned patients by transferring strips of their own collagen from another site on their body into their lips—in most cases without the advancement part of the procedure. The case below is an example of the extraordinary.

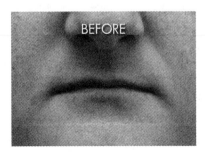 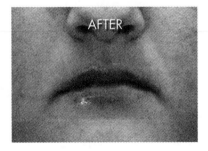

Unlike the hardened, unnatural-feeling lip that results from the insertion of factory-produced enhancers, a patient's own collagen provides a soft, natural texture. In cases where the lips are extremely thin, lip advancement and lip augmentation might be performed at the same time.

As previously mentioned, in lip augmentations, incisions are made at the corners of the mouth and closed with absorbable sutures, which usually dissolve within five to seven days. In lip advancements, incision lines go through the usual maturation process, during which the scar is pink and lumpy for a few weeks and eventually blends into the surrounding tissues once it is totally healed. (Refer to the photographs above.) However, as is the case with any surgical procedure, healing takes time. Most patients agree that, for the long-term results obtained, the additional healing time is well spent.

Some of my patients desire correction of the upper or lower lip only. Most, however, choose to have both enhanced. An important point to remember is that regardless of the treatment methods chosen, after healing is complete, the lower lip should always be *slightly larger* than the upper lip. This is an ideal relationship that Leonardo da Vinci described in the 1600s, yet it has not always found its way into the twenty-first century. If you encounter a person whose lips appear deformed, compare the size of the upper lip with the lower. In most cases, you will find that the operator or injector did not follow Leonardo's criteria of facial proportions.

Either of the lip procedures can be performed in isolation or combined with most of the other surgical procedures discussed in this book. Following any lip surgery, your lips will be swollen and initially appear overly corrected. However, within a couple of weeks, the vast majority of the swelling from the procedure will have subsided. By this point, most patients will be able to return to their work or social activities.

CHAPTER 15

Corrective Surgery for Protruding Ears

One of the most memorable cases I can recall is that of a woman in her early forties who consulted me because she wanted her protruding ears set back closer to her head. She shared with me that when she was eleven years old, she attended a swimming party. When she stepped out of the pool, her hair was wet, and her ears protruded through the soaked strands. One of her classmates screamed, "My God, look at her ears!"

As directed, all who heard this looked at her ears and laughed in unison. It was an experience that was forever implanted in her mind. As long as she was in school with those same classmates, she was known by the nickname "Ears." Of greater import is that when I met her, she had not gone swimming in public since she was eleven years old. However, in anticipation of the appearance of her new ears, she had bought three new bathing suits and looked forward to going swimming in the same pool where the incident had occurred.

You would be surprised to learn how many times a year I hear similar stories from my patients about how the appearance-enhancing surgeries I perform give them the self-confidence they need to engage in public events they once avoided.

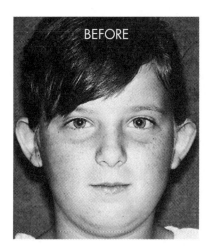
BEFORE

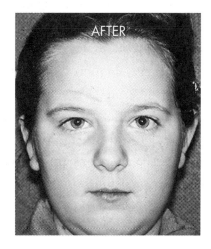
AFTER

Large or protruding ears can be repositioned with a procedure known as otoplasty. Although the procedure does not change the actual size of the ears, it helps them assume a much more natural relationship to the head so that the patient's ears no longer become the center of attention.

As was the case with the patient whose story I shared in the previous paragraphs, abnormally protruding or deformed ears often cause deeper emotional upset than the person's friends or parents generally realize. Because the visual and psychological improvement following the operation is usually dramatic, it is rewarding to the patient, the family, and to the surgeon.

When it comes to how age relates to the dilemma of whether to have your or your child's ears corrected, consider this: by the age of six, a person's ears have reached about 90 percent of their adult size, so little growth of the ears occurs after this time. Because the anterior half of the head develops inside the mother's womb from two sides, rarely are the two ears identical prior to surgery. If they are not identical, chances are there will also be some differences in the two ears after surgery. (See "Facial Analysis" in chapter 13.)

As is the case with large noses and small chins, there is a genetic predisposition to a person having protruding ears. In some families, an entire generation might be skipped. Some family members will have ears that look fairly uniform, but for others, one or usually both ears will protrude to at least some degree. Even if only one ear appears to protrude excessively, it is usually necessary to correct both in order to obtain the desired surgical result.

During embryonic development before birth, everyone's ears project straight out from the head. By the eighth month of gestation, they usually assume a position closer to the head and develop the natural folds and convolutions. In patients whose ears are prominent and lack the usual folds and convolutions, this aspect of the developmental process stopped short of completion.

If addressed during the first week or so following delivery, a baby's deformed ears can often be corrected by applying a custom-made splint that is worn for a several days; however, if the condition is not immediately addressed, the only solution is surgery. For more information on this procedure, consult McCulloughPlasticSurgery.com.

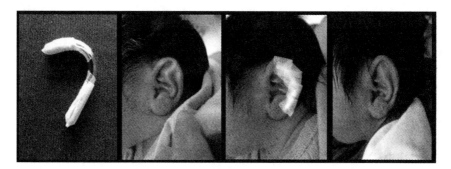

First photo is of an ear splint taylor made by Dr. Yula Indeyeva at the McCollough Plastic Surgery Clinic, second photo is before treatment, third photo is after splint applied by Dr. Yula Indeyeva and last photo is after ear splinting treatment. Photos courtesy of Dr. Yula Indeyeva.

The otoplasty procedure is designed to complete the developmental process by positioning the ears closer to the head and creating the folds that did not develop on their own by placing sutures in the ear cartilages so that they can heal in the desired position.

To avoid classroom teasing and hurtful nicknames, the surgery is preferably performed before a child begins school. However, otoplasty can be performed at any age, just as a person might choose to wear braces to correct the alignment of their teeth at any time in their life.

As each of us ages, our earlobes continue to enlarge with each passing year. With a minor surgical procedure—performed with local anesthesia in a surgeon's office—it is possible to reduce the size of only the earlobes without changing the remainder of the ear. Because earlobes continue to enlarge with aging, earlobe reduction is often performed in conjunction with face-lifting surgery.

When the ear cartilage is thick and strong, it tends to resist being repositioned, and a tuck procedure might be indicated within six to twelve months; however, in my experience, this is an extremely rare occurrence.

CHAPTER 16

Appearance-Enhancing Surgery:

A Condition-Specific Perspective

Regardless of how vigilantly we follow the recommendations in this book, we cannot escape the aging process. However, it is possible to delay the process and address the undesirable sequelae of aging as they occur. This chapter and others that follow are intended to show you how to do so as safely and economically as possible.

As an appearance-enhancement surgeon, when I am interviewed by a member of the media, the question I'm most frequently asked is, "Doctor, can you share with our audience what is *new* in your profession?"

In response, I usually reply, "I'll spend as much time discussing what's new as you wish, as long as you will allow me equal time to discuss the procedures and products that are tried, tested, and true."

My response is not intended to create contentious dialogue between the interviewer and myself but to emphasize a point media circles often overlook: what's *new* is not always what's *best*. "Too good to be true" procedures and products lure many unsuspecting patients into subjecting themselves to risks and spending money that might not produce the results advertised. In that regard, the only time-tested remedy for correcting the signs of aging with any degree of permanency is age-reversing surgery.

Surgery turns back the clock; it does not stop the aging process. In fact, no operation or commercially produced product can permanently prevent aging. But the individual who has undergone surgery to reverse the signs of aging should never again appear as old as they might have if the operation had not been performed. With age-reversing surgery, it is as though one's appearance is moved several years back on the conveyor belt of time. The number of years is directly related to the procedures performed and the surgeon who performs them. In short, there is no one-size-fits-all facial rejuvenation plan. If the surgeon is experienced and uses that experience to recommend the appropriate surgery for the conditions at hand, the patient could appear as much as ten to fifteen years younger. However, the moment the surgeon places the last suture in the operating room, the aging process continues.

A fact to keep in mind is that aged skin removed at the time of a facelift, eyelid surgery, breast lifting, or tummy tuck is gone forever. Skin that remains, however, continues to age at a rate that is, to a large extent, dependent upon other factors I address in this book, such as the patient's lifestyle habits and whether they follow up with a professionally overseen skin-care and weight-management program.

Common Misconceptions

Much has been written in the lay press about appearance-enhancement procedures and products offered by nonphysicians. In an attempt to write something new or to sensationalize the story, half truths published in the media have often led to public misconceptions.

The following are questions I am frequently asked to address by misinformed patients.

How Long Does Plastic Surgery Last?

Many patients believe that once they have one appearance-enhancing surgery, they *must* have another, because if they don't, they will look worse than if they never had the first surgery. This is a myth and has not been my experience or the experience of my like-minded colleagues.

In keeping with the fact that the aging process is not halted by a surgery, it is true that a maintenance minilift (tuck up) at some future date can improve the new signs of aging that appear following the initial surgery. I remind you, however, that excess skin removed at the time of the original surgery is discarded; it is gone forever. The remaining tissues age by the same natural process that caused you to consult an appearance-enhancement surgeon in the first place.

You should also know that surgeons who perform appearance-enhancing surgery do not all have the same training, experience, or mind-set. While it might seem a stretch, imagine that you are going to have your home redecorated. If you were to consult several professionals in the industry, you would likely be presented with a wide variety of choices. The analogy holds true when consulting a professional about enhancing your appearance, regardless of the age at which you choose to do so.

The drawing above appeared in a prominent newspaper in my state. As a newly informed consumer, you can quickly recognize that more than a facelift would be required to obtain the result depicted above. In my opinion, a facelift, a blepharoplasty (eyelid surgery), and a full-face skin-resurfacing procedure combined with a balanced skin-care program might produce the kind of results depicted on the left side of the fictitious patient's face. Other

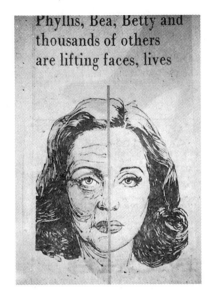

Phyllis, Bea, Betty and thousands of others are lifting faces, lives

surgeons might offer a different treatment plan. So how are you, as a consumer, to know which plan you should agree to? It is the seminal decision every individual in search of the ideal face and body for their age and circumstances must make.

Once the aging process in your face sets in and breakdown of the skin (and structures within and beneath) becomes apparent, the snowball effect seems to come into play. The aging process appears to accelerate. You must understand that the rate of continued aging and sagging is dependent upon a variety of factors that are not under the surgeon's control. Many are of a mental nature, exhibited by the lifestyle that you choose to adopt and live on a daily basis.

Following Plastic Surgery, Will I Still Look Like Me?

The unnatural, stretched, or windblown look frequently seen at the hands of some surgeons is not a result simply of the fact that the patient underwent plastic surgery. Rather, it is a result of how the surgery was performed. It is a result of the surgeon they chose stretching the skin and pulling it backward in an unnatural direction rather than strategically and artfully replacing the sagging tissues into the positions they once occupied.

Recognizing this untoward practice within my profession, I created the condition-specific McCollough Facial Rejuvenation System. Though the system has a long and technical name, it is specifically designed to avoid the overoperated look by performing only as much surgery as is required to address the patient's current conditions—no more, no less. In my system, the sagging tissues are lifted, rather than stretched, and replaced where they were several years previously—in most cases, where they were ten to fifteen years before.

Any elite facial plastic surgeon will demonstrate how their procedures are designed to help safeguard against the justified concern of patients contemplating a facelift or eyelid surgery. But how does a person interested in enhancing their appearance find such a surgeon? The answer to the question is not a simple one. I address it in great detail in my book *The Elite Facial Plastic Surgery Practice*, published by the largest publisher of medical textbooks in the world. To prospective patients and medical colleagues alike, I recommend considering the advice and admonitions I share therein, as well as those shared in this book. Keep in mind that the postoperative result you get is directly related to the mind-set and experience of the surgeon you choose. As recommended in other sections of this book, do the research. If you are not totally comfortable with the first, second, or third surgeon you consult, keep searching. And do not let price be the deciding factor. As is the case with other professions, you generally get what you pay for. That does not necessarily mean that the most expensive surgeon is the surgeon for you, but I'd advise you to be cautious about choosing the least expensive one.

Should I Lose Weight before a Facelift or Tummy Tuck?

This is another question often asked. If you are committed to losing more than twenty pounds, dramatic changes in your face and body will occur. If this amount of weight loss applies to you, I recommend that you postpone surgery until your weight is within eight to ten pounds of your realistic weight goal. I stress *realistic* because it makes no sense to lose thirty pounds only to gain back ten. This yo-yo effect serves only to stretch skin and produce periods of malnutrition.

If, however, you plan to lose only five to ten pounds, the change in your weight will not significantly alter what a facelift, tummy tuck (abdominoplasty), or body liposuction is designed to accomplish. Furthermore, we mind/body/spirit surgeons prefer that our patients be well nourished prior to and after surgery. Crash diets tend to deplete the body of the essential nutrients needed for proper healing and are not recommended. In addition, elite appearance-enhancement practices can also assist you with a personalized weight-management program.

Will Surgery Correct Wrinkled Skin?

Neither surgery nor skin resurfacing can correct wrinkles that occur only during facial expressions. Please reread the preceding sentence and understand that the creases around your eyes produced by smiling (crow's feet), the forehead creases that occur with frowning or lifting your brows, and the vertical lines in your upper lip that occur with puckering are due to the bunching of aging skin whenever the muscles of facial expression are called into action. This is where the group of injectable products known as neuromodulators tends to be helpful. The most common are Botox, Dysport, and Xeomin. These products temporarily paralyze the muscles that create wrinkling with facial expressions. Care must be exercised when using neuromodulators around the mouth. Inexperienced injectors might cause drooling that can last for weeks or months. Once again, the central theme I have emphasized throughout this book applies: *experience counts!* Your local day spa or beauty salon suddenly offering injectable therapies should serve as a warning. Make sure the injector with whom they have become affiliated is board certified in a specialty that traditionally trains and certifies surgeons for aesthetic procedures and experienced in the treatments you are considering.

None of the surgical procedures discussed in this book are designed to eliminate wrinkling that occurs only with activating the muscles of facial expression. For wrinkles and creases that are present at rest, I recommend skin-resurfacing procedures (chemical peeling, laser, or dermabrasion.) For wrinkles that occur only when the muscles of facial expression are engaged, I recommend neuromodulators. Level 2 and 3 skin resurfacing procedures are rarely performed on patients of color.

Following Skin-Rejuvenation Procedures, Is Sun Exposure Allowed?

Prospective patients who have not read my practice-specific consumer information book (*The Appearance Factor*) are often misinformed about the long-term restriction of activities following a skin-resurfacing procedure. From friends, family, and misled posts on the internet, they have heard that once they have undergone a level 2 or 3 peel, dermabrasion, or laser procedure performed by an appearance-enhancement surgeon, they can never enjoy the sun again. Here I stress the surgeon component, because many day spas and nonsurgical clinics offer superficial (level 1) peels that do not penetrate deeply enough into a patient's skin to stimulate the deeper layers of collagen. These superficial peels only temporarily *polish* the skin for a couple of weeks, in the same manner that furniture polish causes a wooden surface to shine. But they are incapable of removing the wrinkles of aging.

Although it is important to avoid excessive sun exposure and to use sunscreen products for several months after level 2 and level 3 peels, dermabrasions, and laser treatments, sun exposure that is sensible and protected is allowed after a few weeks or when the pink color of healing skin has returned to its natural color. It simply takes time for the baby-like new skin created by level 2 and level 3 resurfacing procedures to build up a natural resistance to sun and wind, just as your skin did in the earliest months and years of your life.

Whether or not you have undergone a skin-rejuvenation procedure, I recommend sunscreen products for prolonged exposure, cradle to grave.

However, following a skin-resurfacing procedure, it is wise not to use any topically applied product until your surgeon instructs you to do so. Many such products contain preservatives and active ingredients that can irritate newly rejuvenated skin. Experienced skin-care experts can assist you with a program designed to protect and preserve the more youthful skin achieved through the professionally performed skin-resurfacing procedures I address in this book.

Following Appearance-Enhancing Procedures, When Will I Be Presentable?

It stands to reason that different individuals respond to the same treatment in different ways. The following addresses many of the conditions that are common to the population at large.

Some degree of swelling follows any surgical procedure, including level 2 and level 3 skin-resurfacing procedures. The swelling and tightness are due to the new tissue fluids strategically brought into the area by your body to promote healing. Increased blood supply to the region is responsible for the pink color of the skin and for some of the discoloration (bruising) associated with surgery and skin-resurfacing procedures. When these essential healing fluids are no longer required, the tissues release them into the bloodstream, and the color of the skin in the treated areas usually returns to a more natural color.

If and when you choose to undergo appearance-enhancement procedures, you must be willing to accept temporary swelling, tightness, and discoloration, which are a natural part of the healing process. Although usually visually disconcerting, these conditions represent a negligible inconvenience for the physical and psychological improvement most people experience when the healing process has run its course.

Here, I insert a caveat that arises from more than four decades of performing appearance-enhancement procedures: to a great extent, how quickly any patient heals from procedures depends upon how carefully they adhere to the doctor's orders prior to and after treatment.

When an incision is made through the full thickness of the skin, that incision can only heal by producing a scar. It is nature's way of mending the two severed edges together. In the hands of elite surgeons, every attempt is made to have the scars heal as narrowly and smoothly as possible. Whenever possible, the placement of surgically created scars is designed to camouflage them in natural facial folds and creases or hide them within or at the edges of hairlines. Facelift incisions can be made so that hair will actually grow through the scar, thereby making it even less noticeable.

During the initial healing period following any surgical procedure, scars will appear pink, somewhat swollen, and lumpy. The pink color is due to the increased blood supply that your body directs into the area—a process instilled at the time of our creation to promote healing. As healing progresses and scars become mature, they usually become less conspicuous; the pink discoloration disappears, and they flatten and blend into the surrounding tissues. In most cases, scars produced by elite surgeons eventually become barely visible to the casual observer. At any rate, properly applied cosmetics and hair styling after the operation can help camouflage them. In addition, permanent makeup can be placed within the scar to have it match the surrounding skin.

How quickly the healing process runs its course depends as much on the patient's compliance with the venerable principles of healings as with the surgeon's skills. In keeping with the theme of this book, people who have undergone appearance-enhancing surgery can give themselves the best chance to heal quickly and obtain the best possible result by adhering to the recommendations provided by their surgeon and their staff—assuming that such instructions are, in fact, provided. Believe it or not, many providers of appearance-enhancement procedures do not provide written postoperative instructions to their patients. You should ask any provider you're considering to provide you with any instructions that they would give you, and you should ask days in advance of undergoing the procedures they recommend.

Patients who have undergone skin-resurfacing procedures (laser, peeling, or dermabrasion) and who live or recover in coastal areas are subject to the detrimental effects of the salty winds coming off the ocean or gulf. This factor, combined with additional sun exposure, makes patients recovering in such regions more subject to prolonged redness and irritation posttreatment.

Regardless of geography, absolute compliance with posttreatment instructions is the best way to ensure rapid healing and happier outcomes. If, however, skin-resurfacing procedures have not been performed at the time of other rejuvenating procedures, patients may be out of doors— even on the beach and on boats—within a few days.

The much-feared type of scar called a keloid is extremely rare on the face. Certainly, however, some people are more prone to scarring than others, especially those whose ancestors were born in African nations.

Following appearance-enhancing surgery, most patients resume their preoperative routine within one to two weeks. Patients who undergo skin-resurfacing procedures should allow three weeks. At that point, mineral powder makeup and creative hairstyling are allowed for camouflaging some of the residual signs of healing. A professional aesthetician or cosmetologist can also assist with makeup and hairstyle counseling. However, for patients who have undergone level 2 or level 3 skin-resurfacing procedures, exposure to the chemicals in hair and nail salons can create irritation of treated areas, much like a newborn baby can develop a diaper rash.

A systematic posttreatment skin-care program administered by a trained aesthetician in concert with an appearance-enhancement surgeon can not only speed up the healing process but also help maintain the desired appearance of healthier, happier skin for years to come. With this thought in mind, I strongly recommend that my patients consult with a medical aesthetician who has a professional relationship with me and my staff about the various programs and products that can further enhance the surgical procedures performed.

Will I Be Happier after Undergoing Appearance-Enhancement Surgery?

In my experience, most of my patients are elated with the outcome of their appearance-enhancing procedures. However, an operation alone is incapable of turning an unhappy person into a happy person. Your own attitude toward your special set of circumstances is the key that unlocks the gateways to happiness. It is important not only that you recognize this fact but that your prospective surgeon does as well.

Neither you nor your surgeon should expect plastic surgery to solve personal, domestic, or professional problems. Nor should you seek universal approval from family, friends, or acquaintances before or after surgery. Undergoing appearance-enhancing surgery is a personal choice based upon realistic expectations and mutual trust between you and your surgeon. In uncomplicated cases, patients are usually glad they underwent the surgery and recommend similar surgical procedures to friends and family.

Although I refer to the average case throughout this book, each patient's experience is unique. The final outcome depends upon myriad factors, risk, and imponderables. Should you have questions after surgery, we urge you to contact the surgeon who performed the procedures first. If, after doing so, you are not satisfied, contact another life-enhancement professional.

Is It Possible to Have Multiple Procedures Performed at the Same Time?

The answer is a resounding yes! It is possible for you to have several procedures performed during the same operation. Your health, the types of procedures to be performed, and the schedules of the surgeons might determine the extent of the surgery recommended. Convenience and financial savings generally come into play when multiple procedures are performed at the same time. In addition, in the time during which you recover from one procedure, you could be recovering from multiple procedures. You might be surprised to learn how many family members and friends choose to have surgery at the same time, including husbands and wives.

It is important to remember that the aging process continues to move forward after surgery and that your chronological and biological clocks keep ticking. In time, your appearance will catch up to your original position on the conveyor belt of time. However, had age-defying surgery not been performed, you would have been farther down the line on that proverbial conveyor belt, and your appearance would have reflected that fact. In that regard, a surgical facial rejuvenation procedure lasts forever, as you will always appear younger than you would had you not undergone the initial procedure and further procedures designed to help maintain a youthful appearance.

These irrefutable facts of nature must be understood and accepted by patients and surgeons alike. The good news is that once you have undergone the procedures I recommend in this book, the procedures performed to maintain the results are less extensive and less expensive. This means that you can maintain a more youthful appearance for as long as you remain healthy. The inexorable connection between these two factors is why I include them in this book. Your task is to learn how to take care of your body, mind, and soul and to apply those principles to an everyday lifestyle. My task—and that of my colleagues—is to assist you in becoming the person of your dreams for years to come.

CHAPTER 17

A More Youthful Face:

Before You Consent to Altering It

By now, you have realized that facial rejuvenation entails a wide variety of procedures and products. In this chapter, we explore the most commonly recommended surgical procedures.

"Facelift" is often used as a catchall term when referring to a facial rejuvenation makeover. However, a facelift is only part of the plan. The procedure recreates the firm, smooth face of youth in the neck, cheeks, and forehead. However, it does not address the sagging and bulging tissues around the eyes; nor does it remove wrinkles embedded in the skin of the face or address thinning lips.

I'd like to share with you a fact of which I have constantly reminded my appearance-enhancement colleagues, through continuing educational conferences, scientific articles in plastic surgery journals, and textbooks: not all faces are the same. Likewise, not all facelifts (or facial rejuvenation plans) are the same—nor should they be! Furthermore, the same face is a different face at different ages. The facial rejuvenation you might require at the age of forty-five is a different plan than you will need at age sixty-five or seventy-five. Yes, as long as you remain in good health (through many of the recommendations I offer throughout this book), you are a candidate for rejuvenating surgery well into your years. You might be surprised to learn that I have patients in their eighties return for what one of them calls minor "tweaks."

The point I wish to make is that not all faces should undergo the same procedures. Your treatment plan should be personalized to meet the specific conditions present in your face and the goals that you have in mind. Unfortunately, some commercialized assembly-line face-lifting procedures fall under the "one size fits all" ideology—an ideology that more often than not leads to disappointment and money not wisely invested. Some surgeons have been trained to perform the facelift procedure in only one way. In that regard, face lifting is subject to the age-old adage that if all one has is a hammer, everything looks like a nail. When it comes to having the right procedure for you performed at the right time in your life by the right surgeon, you—the consumer—must be your own advocate and make sure that your face is not looked upon as a nail by a surgeon whose training and experience is limited. You should be assured that the surgeon you consult is planning to perform the combination of operations called for in your case, not the operations that they *routinely* perform. Hopefully, this book will encourage you to take advantage of a gift you already have: free will—the ability to choose your destiny from a plethora of alternatives. When you exercise that gift by doing your research and asking your prospective surgeon the hard questions, you immediately increase your chances of becoming the best you possible.

Arm yourself with the knowledge that facial plastic surgery is very much an art form and should be tailored to a specific set of circumstances by an experienced surgeon to meet *your* individual needs. This will improve your chances of obtaining the appearance-enhancing results you desire. The case presented in the photographs below makes the point.

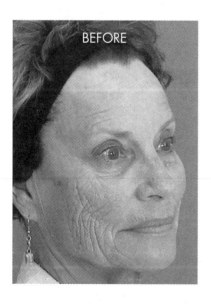
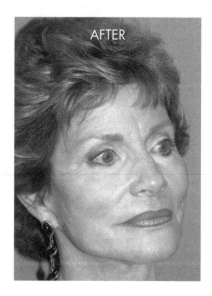

Because of the specific conditions her face exemplified, this patient underwent upper and lower blepharoplasty and face lifting. Several months later, she underwent full-face resurfacing with a chemical peel and dermabrasion to remove deep facial wrinkles. Hers is an example of a comprehensive and condition-specific facial rejuvenation plan.

Prior to undergoing surgery, this patient's face was not the same as it had been when she was twenty years younger, which meant that her treatment plan was different than it would have been had she consulted me at that time in her life. Irrefutably, our faces change with every passing year. In our late thirties or early forties, the tissues of the brows, cheeks, and neck began to descend from their more youthful positions, thereby creating a tired look. Alternating ridges and valleys create shadows in our faces, and tissues begin to hang below our jawlines and under our chins. With each passing year, these conditions worsen until we exhibit the undesirable characteristics of aging. However, we do not have to live with these conditions. It is possible for us to both prevent these conditions and to correct them as they occur.

Reversing the undesirable signs of aging is one part of the gift that you are capable of giving yourself. Maintaining a youthful appearance is the other part. The youthful maintenance approach that I recommend for my patients addresses the ever-mounting signs of aging so that the patients who adopt a preventative maintenance policy appear never to age. At the other end of the spectrum, the rejuvenation approach to creating a more youthful face addresses the conditions of aging after they have occurred. Both approaches are equally effective. However, armed with the information you'll need to make an informed decision, you can make better decisions and serve as your own advocate.

The bottom line is that surgery—combined with many of the other measures addressed in this book, including professional skin care, healthy nutrition, and a personalized fitness program—can help you either retain or regain a youthful and vibrant face and body well into your advancing years.

When Is Facial Plastic Surgery Indicated?

"Am I ready for procedures and products proven to be effective in the rejuvenation process?" This question is often asked in my practice. The best way I can answer is to say that when slack in the skin of the face and neck or bulging around the eyes is no longer a temporary condition that is relieved by rest or by reducing your salt or yeast intake—or when these signs become increasingly difficult to camouflage with cosmetics—then it's time to give yourself the face that your mind's eye sees yourself having again. When you exercise that gift, your chronological age becomes much less relevant in the grand schemes of things. When you begin to appear younger, healthier, and more vibrant, the people you encounter will begin to look at you differently. Your appeal index rises. Doors of opportunity begin to swing open and to open more widely. These are documentable facts, not theory. I see them played out on a daily basis.

As the lifespan lengthens in modern America, most people feel vigorous and energetic long after their appearance begins to deteriorate as a result of advancing years. Furthermore, because it has a direct effect on self-esteem, the onset of aging plays an important part in the personal and financial well-being of men and women like you. I'd be willing to bet that you know people whose employment opportunities have been limited or curtailed because they look old or unhealthy, even though they might be more capable and competent than younger individuals. Perhaps, like the woman whose story was shared in chapter 1 of this book, you have experienced similar situations.

The revelations I set forth are not limited to the twenty-first century. For hundreds of years, experts have confirmed that favors are granted to beautiful or handsome people. In Buffington's *Your Behavior Is Showing: Forty Prescriptions for Understanding and Liking Yourself*, the doctor concluded that the benefits of good looks transcend the generational gap. Buffington also concluded that good looks "affect school grades, enhance the probability of prosperity, determine who will be our friends, and shorten stays in mental hospitals."[7]

---

7. Buffington, *Your Behavior Is Showing*.

The appearance of aging also imposes certain limitations when it comes to one's social interests and circle of friends and associates. Finally, the emotional impact of looking older than one feels can become an inhibitor to seeking new opportunities.

When it comes to rejuvenating the mind, body, and spirit, two schools of thought exist. One suggests preserving one's youth and beauty by having the undesirable signs of aging addressed as they occur. The other suggests waiting until the aging process has erased both and then turning to measures that recapture them. In short, preventive maintenance versus restoration.

If you wish to remain looking younger throughout your life, it is possible for the appearance-enhancement surgeon you choose to perform a continuing series of relatively minor cosmetic procedures as each of the undesirable changes of aging makes its appearance. With such a maintenance program, you can be kept looking younger than your chronological age throughout the years, and long-term friends and associates will be apt to remark that you don't seem to grow older.

Today, more and more people are choosing the preventive-maintenance route. But if you are among those who didn't start such a maintenance program when you were younger, it's not too late. Appearance-enhancing professionals can develop a rejuvenation program to help bring out a better you and help you look as young and as well as you feel.

Why Our Faces and Necks Droop and Sag

The physical and mental changes associated with aging do not occur all at once. That's why we refer to aging as a process. The changes we see in our mirrors and experience in our ability to perform the duties expected by ourselves and by others happen in a slow, progressive manner and involve all components of the face, mind, and body.

Each of us is a similar yet unique creation. Yet we age at different rates—and in seven-year cycles. Even though the elusive Fountain of Youth has not yet been discovered, several factors can shorten the seven-year process. My patients frequently share with me that they became aware of the undesirable signs of aging during their forties, occasionally sooner. They often comment that it seems as though they were holding up well and then seemed to age almost overnight, especially following prolonged stress and the extreme hormonal changes that occur within the body during those periods.

Aging is not an isolated phenomenon. It affects all body parts and organs. The skull becomes smaller. In certain areas, fat is absorbed. In other areas, fat accumulates, clumps, or sags. Clumped fat cells are often referred to as cellulite.

In all areas of the body, you might notice that your skin loses its elasticity and has no alternative other than to yield to the forces of gravity. In short, the envelope of skin becomes larger than its contents. In the face and neck, this phenomenon results in changes including deepening of the lines of facial expression in the forehead and at the sides of the mouth, sagging of the eyebrows (which causes the eyes to appear smaller), the formation of crow's feet at the corners of the eyes, the appearance of pouches or jowls along the jawline, and, of course, the appearance of the well-known "double chin" in your neck. In other parts of the body, both men and women notice that their breasts sag. The skin in the abdomen laps over the belt line, the buttocks wither and droop, and the skin of the arms and legs becomes irregular and floppy.

At the same time, other degenerative changes occur. In addition to sagging, the skin becomes wrinkled, thinner, and displays brown spots or precancerous conditions. The face becomes etched with wrinkles, especially the faces of those repetitively exposed without protection to the sun and wind. Keep in mind that cold, salty air, while a lesser factor than sun exposure, also wreaks havoc on your skin's appearance and health.

With aging, the muscles and tissues around your eyes eventually lose some of their tone, such that a portion of the fat normally located inside the orbit around the eye bulges forward, or herniates, to produce the commonly seen bags or pouches. Premature development of these conditions is often visible in younger people, especially those who suffer from allergies.

Dark circles underneath the eyes might be a result of a shadowing effect caused by bulges on either side where your lower eyelids meet your cheeks. Even in adults, these bulges could be caused by allergies and fluid collection from excessive salt and yeast intake in your diet. Yes—yeast-containing foods and drinks, such as bread, cookies, cake, beer, wine, and liquor, contain yeast and might contribute to fluid retention throughout your body.

Finally, because of thinning of the gums and absorption of fat and thinning of the muscles in the upper lip, the tip of the nose drops, causing it to appear larger and longer. As the tip of the nose drops, breathing can become impaired.

And do not forget that earlobes continue to enlarge with age. Refining the nose and reducing the size of earlobes, with or without face lifting and eyelid surgery, can have a dramatic and lasting effect on reversing the telltale signs of aging. (See photographs below.)

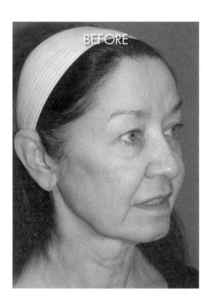
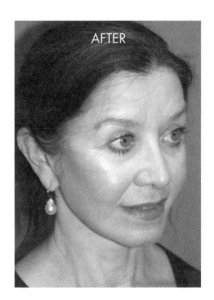

To see what has happened to your face, you need only to study a childhood photograph or any child's face. Compare the physical characteristics that exemplify youth (fuller lips, larger eyes, arched eyebrows, smoother skin, and a shorter nose) and realize that carefully planned and skillfully executed plastic surgery can help you look younger than your chronological age.

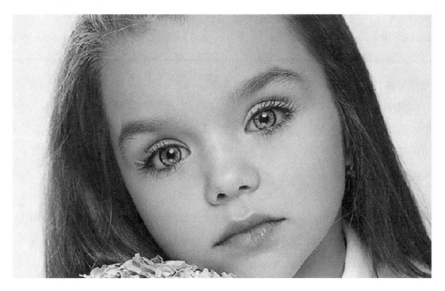

With the information presented above, I trust that you are becoming a better-informed consumer of appearance-enhancing therapies and that you better understand why, as a unique individual, you present a different set of problems and challenges than anyone else. Consequently, the corrective procedures indicated for you might be different than those indicated for anyone else you know, such as your siblings. For example, when it comes to facial rejuvenation, at one stage of your life you might require only elevation of sagging eyebrows or improvement in the eyelids. You might need only to correct an early double chin with liposuction. On the other hand, a partial or complete face and neck lift accompanied by a skin-resurfacing procedure might be called for when you exhibit the advanced stages of the aging process. (See photographs below.) The same is true with the breasts, abdomens, legs, and arms of both women and men.

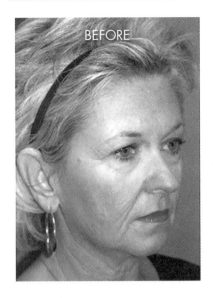
BEFORE

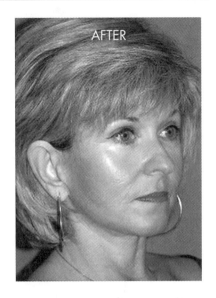
AFTER

If your skin is weather beaten in appearance or is etched with deep wrinkles, one of the skin-resurfacing procedures discussed in a future chapter (chemical face peel, dermabrasion, or laser resurfacing) might provide the enhancement you are seeking.

A good truth for you to remember is that a facelift, blepharoplasty, or submental liposuction improves sags and bulges. Surgical skin-rejuvenation procedures (level 2 and 3 laser, dermabrasion, and peeling) improve wrinkles, and fillers (your own collagen and sometimes fat) improve deeper facial creases. Beginning in chapter 29, I address rejuvenation of body parts and areas below the neck.

Prevention or Rejuvenation? Where You Are in the Process

If you are committed to looking in the mirror and seeing the face of your dreams, there are two acceptable schools of thought. Some experts believe that as soon as undesirable signs of aging appear, they should be corrected. Thus, you will never appear as old as your chronological age would suggest. The majority of entertainment personalities and public figures who have enjoyed long careers in the industry followed this principle of preventative maintenance. They never allowed themselves to look old. Some, however, waited too long and then were taken to the extreme by surgeons who did not apply a condition-specific approach to the rejuvenation plan they recommended and carried out. As a result, some of these high-profile individuals barely resemble themselves following plastic surgery and the overuse of fillers. This "plastic" or "windblown" appearance can—and should—be avoided. It is a matter of the surgeon recommending and performing techniques that create a natural appearance at every age. It is also a result of the fact that many of these high-profile individuals were not appropriately armed with the information with which you are being provided. They did not know how to become their own advocate and ask the questions that you know to ask if and when you choose to undergo appearance-enhancing surgery.

Those who wait until the signs of aging are beyond maintenance frequently regret not having had surgery done earlier so that they could have enjoyed their more youthful look longer.

In the 1990s, comedian Phyllis Diller announced her plastic surgery makeover to the entire world. But she might as well have gone public with her makeover; she experienced such a dramatic improvement in her appearance that even the least informed segment of the public would have guessed she had undergone extensive plastic surgery. Most people would rather keep the fact that they have had surgery more private than she did. Today, with a well-conceived—and well-performed—maintenance program, it is possible to keep the world guessing. And after all, isn't that what most of us want?

As I have long pointed out in my writings and lectures, and as fellow appearance-enhancement physicians and surgeons are beginning to recognize, the motivation for any human being to look their best is well placed. Doing so should be considered an investment in yourself—an inestimable gift that you can choose to give to yourself.

If you take pride in your health, pay attention to your clothing, grooming, and overall personal appearance, and realize that exercise and proper nutrition can keep the rest of your body toned and looking more youthful than its chronological years, then you can give yourself a big pat on the back. You are fulfilling the purpose of your creation. You are exercising the gift known as free will to become the best version of yourself that you can be—the you of your dreams.

Regardless of what you might read or hear elsewhere, as it stands at the time of this writing, nothing short of surgery can help an aging face maintain as youthful an appearance. Too-good-to-be-true remedies such as facial exercises, electrical stimulation, needling, or "facelifts in a jar" enhance the quality and texture of the skin and might provide some degree of toning, but none of these procedures can achieve the results obtained through well-conceived and skillfully performed surgery and skin-resurfacing procedures. Nonsurgical alternatives should be considered *in addition to* rather than *in lieu of* treatments.

Here are the facts that you should keep at the forefront of your mind. Injectable fillers dissolve within weeks to months, requiring multiple treatments, and are not without their own set of complications. Except in extenuating circumstances (health conditions that would preclude surgery and upcoming events that do not allow the appropriate time frame to heal from surgery), I recommend more predictable—and lasting—alternatives. Once again, conventional wisdom prevails. Quick fixes generally lead to quick returns of the condition treated, requiring ongoing treatments and more money spent.

Because I am familiar with the mind-set and practices of the vast majority of my colleagues, I can make the following statement without reservation: elite appearance-enhancement surgeons evaluate each patient and their specific conditions and recommend the most effective treatment available. This group of mainstream surgeons is constantly investigating procedures and techniques designed to provide the best result with the least risks for the longest period of time feasible. If and when promising alternatives to surgery and therapeutic skin resurfacing come along, we will be the first to bring these alternatives to your attention.

Allow me to share an example of how the last statement holds true. For treating wrinkles of the face, I was trained to perform therapeutic (levels 2 and 3) chemical peeling. For treating facial scarring (especially that produced by uncontrolled acne), I was trained to perform levels 2 and 3 dermabrasion. Then, in the early 1990s, laser skin resurfacing came on the scene. After being convinced by the manufacturers and marketers that laser resurfacing was going to replace chemical peeling and dermabrasion, I opened the first laser center in the state of Alabama.

For the next five years, I stopped performing chemical peels and dermabrasion; however, after reviewing the long-term results, I came to the conclusion that lasers were not better than the methods in which I had been trained. So, I did what any results-oriented appearance-enhancement surgeon would do: I abandoned laser therapy for skin rejuvenation and returned to performing chemical peels and dermabrasion. It is a practice that, some twenty-five years later, I continue to follow.

In a future chapter, I address some of the other conditions of the face and body that I have determined are best treated with various types of lasers and related devices.

So, now we come full circle back to the question posed at the beginning of this chapter. *When* is the time to consider appearance-enhancing surgery? The answer you may have been waiting for is this: when the face you see in the mirror does not match the person you feel yourself to be—the person you imagine yourself to be. That is when you might want to consider consulting an elite facial plastic surgeon. By now, you know that not everyone seeking plastic surgery is an acceptable candidate. Elite appearance-enhancing surgeons usually require preoperative screening in the form of laboratory tests and a note from your personal physician indicating that you are an acceptable risk to undergo the procedures recommended by your surgeon. If your surgeon does not require medical clearance, I would recommend that you, as your best advocate, exercise your prerogative and seek one on your own accord. Appearance-enhancing surgery is elective surgery. Both you and your surgeon should want to know whether there are any underlying health problems that could cause problems during or after surgery.

You should also know that responsible and ethical surgeons advise against elective surgery in patients who have been diagnosed with serious diseases, who are too obese, who we think have unrealistic expectations or improper motivation, who cannot accept improvement—rather than perfection—as the goal, who refuse to comply with our treatment recommendations, or who insist on debating the postoperative care instructions we recommend.

I venture to say that, as a potential consumer of appearance- and health-enhancing procedures and products, you are already better informed than the segment of society that has not been exposed to the information and admonitions shared in this book. Even so, I urge you to keep reading. We have only scratched the surface of the life-enhancement alternatives that are available to you and others who are committed to seeing the person of their dreams come into view.

CHAPTER 18

Sagging and Aging Eyelids:

The Corrective Procedure Known as Blepharoplasty

Our eyelids have both functional and aesthetic purposes. On the functional side of the equation, they are intended to protect our eyeballs. On the aesthetic side, they provide an anatomical frame around the part of the eyeball that others see.

In light of those facts, my interest in correcting conditions of and around the eyelids arose from a moonlighting job (or what I preferred to call a "beyond the core-curriculum experience") I held during my last two years of medical school. On alternating evenings after completing my duties at UAB's university hospital, I walked two blocks west to the Eye Foundation Hospital (EFH), where I proceeded to perform preoperative histories and physicals on patients who were scheduled to undergo surgery on their eyes and the surrounding structures the following morning.

The experience was enlightening enough that I seriously considered oculoplastic surgery as a career. That option was offered to me by the founder of the EFH, Dr. Alston Callahan, who also wrote the first textbook on the subject. However, because I wanted to perform plastic and reconstructive surgery beyond the eyelids and brows, I chose to expand my training and skills into the face, nose, head, and neck. Nevertheless, the two years I spent assisting eye surgeons in preparing their patients for surgery provided insight and experiences that give me a unique perspective on the treatment of conditions in this region of the face and body. Those experiences are also part of the broad-based foundation I use in order to provide the following information and admonitions.

Drooping, heavy tissues around the eyes can be removed with an upper- and lower-lid plastic procedure (blepharoplasty) and improve the "tired look" that many of my patients want corrected. The before and after photographs below show only one of the more than seven thousand patients whose eyelids I have been honored to correct.

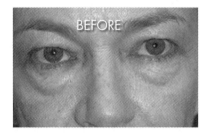 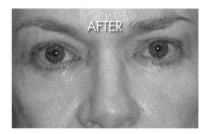

Here are the facts that underlie the procedures I recommend in this book and when I stand behind my patients in front of a three-way mirror during an official consultation. From a functional and appearance-enhancing perspective, each of us has four eyelids—two upper lids and two lower lids. As the aging process progresses, we become plagued by wrinkles, loose skin, and bulges in those areas of our faces. These conditions can also occur as a result of hereditary factors and health-related conditions such as thyroid disease, kidney failure, allergies, and excessive salt and yeast intake.

Not unlike hernias in other parts of the human body, pouches or bags of the upper and lower lids are generally due to herniations of fat that, in a youthful and totally healthy body, are localized within the eye socket. These fatty protrusions can be surgically removed by making incisions either inside the eyelid or in a wrinkle line just beyond the eyelashes. In this region of our bodies, unwanted and unattractive fat is removed under direct vision rather than by liposuction.

Fatty pouches are often seen in the twenty- to thirty-year-old age group of our society—and sometimes in those younger—and can be addressed by a facial or oculoplastic surgeon whenever the condition arises.

From the functional perspective of health and well-being, excess skin in the upper eyelid often causes a feeling of heaviness, especially late in the day, and in extreme cases creates a hooding effect that obstructs your ability to see objects to your sides. In both cases, there is little rationale for waiting for some arbitrary date on a calendar before having this trouble-some condition surgically corrected. (See photographs below.)

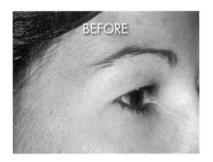
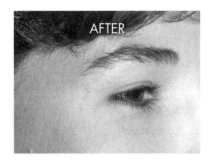

Regardless of your chronological age, if you are experiencing any of these signs and symptoms, you should know that upper-lid surgery is usually done at the same time as lower-lid surgery, but either can be done as an isolated procedure. In both cases, under sedation and local anesthesia, the excess skin and fat are removed, and the incision sites (if required) are closed with delicate sutures. As a result—assuming that your surgeon applies the principles that I was taught and have since paid forward—once your healing process has run its course, your incisions will be visible only with magnification, if at all.

Plastic surgery of the upper or lower eyelid may be done with or without a facelift, brow lift, or other appearance-enhancing surgery.

No-Scar Lower-Lid Surgery: Transconjunctival Blepharoplasty

If you are considering surgical correction in any area of your body, you must keep the following truism at the forefront of your decision-making process. Everything in life—including appearance-enhancing surgery—is a matter of exchanging one condition for another. If herniated fat produces bags or bulges in your lower lid but you do not have loose skin or wrinkles in that region of your face, the fat can be removed without making an incision in your skin. It is made *behind* your lower lid, thereby eliminating the possibility of a scar, even though the incision itself is negligible.

In keeping with the principle of exchange described in the preceding paragraph, it is not possible to remove loose skin or sagging wrinkles when the behind-the-eyelid technique is used. However, level 2 skin resurfacing (laser, peeling, or dermabrasion) can be performed at the same time (and in some cases when outside incisions are required) in order to minimize fine wrinkles. In some cases, in order to obtain the best possible result, it is necessary to include both incisional surgery and chemical peeling.

Classic Lower-Lid Blepharoplasty

In my practice, the traditional lower-lid rejuvenation procedure is performed by making an incision in the first wrinkle line below the lower lashes. I then elevate the skin and muscle so that the fatty pouches or hernias can be identified. Once herniated fat is removed, excess skin is trimmed and discarded.

Small, delicate sutures are used to close the lower-lid incisions. Because the skin at the outer corners of the eye is thicker than that adjacent to the lashes, it usually takes a bit longer for the outer part of the incision to soften and flatten. Sometimes, cortisone injections can speed the healing process along. However, with the passage of time, the incision lines of the upper and lower lids will be naturally camouflaged. In my experience, when patients return several years later for "tuck up" procedures, even though I know where I made the original incisions, I am unable to find them.

As a rule, undesirable eyelid conditions tend to occur at earlier ages in men than in women. Surgical correction of these conditions is usually associated with minor recovery restrictions; therefore, patients can usually return to routine living and work activities after a few days, especially when cosmetics and sunglasses are used.

When wrinkling of the lower lid is pronounced, I recommend skin resurfacing to create further tightening of the skin and improve fine wrinkles or crow's feet. If not performed at the time of the original surgery, a skin-resurfacing, wrinkle-reducing procedure can usually be performed in one of my clinic's postoperative rooms during a follow-up visit.

The hard—and inconvenient—fact is that insurance plans do not cover surgical fees and hospitalization expenses for appearance-enhancing (cosmetic) surgery. Ultimately, it is the company or government agency that provides your health-care coverage, not your surgeon or eye doctor, that decides whether a procedure qualifies for the coverage their plan provides. As much as I disagree with this reality, it is one that patients, consultants, and surgeons alike are forced to accept.

In patients who exhibit extreme amounts of overhanging skin of the upper eyelid that clearly impairs their vision, an appearance-enhancing surgeon may (and I emphasize *may*) consult an eye specialist prior to surgery. If the visual field examination demonstrates any impairment of vision as a result of overhanging upper-eyelid skin, a portion of the fees for "functional" upper-lid surgery may be filed to the patient's medical insurance provider, including Medicare. That being said, you should know that even with all the required information, it is getting more and more difficult to convince insurance companies to cover the costs of upper-eyelid surgery, even when functional conditions are clearly present.

I have yet to encounter a case where excess skin and fat in the lower lid impaired one's vision; however, if it were necessary to perform a procedure to support a lax or drooping lower lid (as a result of an age-related weakening of the anatomical lower lid known as a "hammock complex"), as stressed in previous paragraphs, insurance might pay some of the costs for this portion of the lower-lid operation. Please notice that I emphasize the words *might* and *some*. As a duly informed patient, you should enter the process of having the excess skin and fat of your eyelids addressed with the understanding that even though your vision is impaired, you—not your insurance provider—are responsible for the costs incurred.

Sadly, I and my fellow appearance- and health-enhancing colleagues have experienced self-serving practices among health-plan insurance carriers—practices that should be called into question. More often than not, insurance companies *automatically* deny claims for eyelid-related surgery and resort to what seems to be a never-ending series of delay tactics. Only after repeat filings and pressure exerted upon the company by the patient (or the corporation that pays the patient's premiums) do health-care insurance companies negotiate a settlement amount—if ever. And when they do, the amount reimbursed rarely meets the amount submitted. In fact, third-party payers pay only pennies on the dollar, if anything, to the providers of the services rendered. This false flag scenario was masterfully played out in the movie *The Rainmaker*, based upon a John Grisham book by the same name. If you have not seen the movie, or if it has been a while since you did, I recommend you watch it again. As you do, I recommend that you connect the information provided in this book with the storyline of Grisham's book. And remember that Grisham is a lawyer.

As was dramatized in the Grisham story, I have noticed that this reject-and-delay tactic has become an ever-mounting practice among insurance providers. I raise this issue here because the "buyer beware" admonitions I offer throughout this book apply to all surgeries and procedures, especially those designed to enhance your appearance or the function of the parts of your anatomy.

In addition, if you choose to explore plastic or reconstructive surgery of the eyelid, you should advise your surgeon of any history of eye diseases or history of visual problems so that they can take them into consideration or have them evaluated.

Throughout my career, I have recommended that patients have an eye examination conducted by an eye specialist prior to undergoing eyelid surgery. This safeguard is suggested by elite appearance-enhancement surgeons to ensure that the patient does not have an underlying medical condition related to their eyes. I also ask that my patient's eye doctor send a report of their findings to me—as well as to my patient's insurance carrier—prior to performing the surgery in question. As your own health-care advocate, if the surgeon you are considering does not require such an examination and report, I recommend that you take it upon yourself to see that one be performed.

The Eyebrow Factor

In some of my patients, the curtain of skin hanging from the upper eyelid can be partially due to sagging of the eyebrows. In such cases, it might be necessary to advise elevation and support of the brows and forehead at the same time that the upper-lid surgery is performed. (See chapter 19.) I recommend that you examine your eyelids and brows in front of a mirror at home prior to consulting a surgeon. Check to see whether they are identical or symmetrical. Rarely do I find that my patient's eyebrows are. It is essential that both you and your surgeon are aware of this fact prior to performing surgery on your upper eyelids.

The Other Bulge

Blepharoplasty is designed to correct conditions found within the confines of the bony rims of the eye socket. The procedure does not correct undesirable conditions in your cheeks and brows; nor does it correct crow's feet at the outer corners of your eyes. Those conditions require outer brow lifting, skin resurfacing, and sometimes neuromodulators such as Botox, Dysport, and Xeomin.

Many of my patients ask me whether lower-lid surgery removes or improves the swollen, puffy areas that sometimes develop *beneath* the lower lid and over the cheekbones. Although the answer is no, I wish it didn't have to be so. These bulges are thought to be caused by uncontrolled fluid accumulation in the tissues of the upper cheeks where the lymphatic channels from the eye and face intersect. They are, in essence, reservoirs of water (a condition called edema). As previously mentioned, they can be exacerbated by total body fluid accumulation, sometimes caused by allergies or by salt and yeast intake.

Direct excision might remove these unwanted tissues. But in my opinion, such a procedure is not indicated unless the fluid accumulations become quite large. The resultant scar is usually imperceptible but sometimes requires dermabrasion at a later time.

While the vast majority of patients who consult me and my colleagues in facial plastic surgery are women in the second or third quarters of their lives, an ever-increasing number of men are also choosing to undergo appearance-enhancement procedures. In addition to correcting the tired look caused by saggy, baggy eyelids and brows—and the associated feelings of inadequacy that accompany the aging process—many men are turning to performance-enhancement medications in order to regain the vitality that they and their partners once enjoyed.

The next chapter addresses a physical change in the faces of men and women that is associated with aging, particularly when it gives an impression of fatigue and of loss of vitality: drooping eyebrows.

CHAPTER 19

Lifting the Aging and Drooping Eyebrow:

The Pros and Cons

In the 1990s, a US Marshal consulted with me about a concern his colleagues expressed on a daily basis. During our preoperative consultation, the man said that when he reported to work each morning, his coworkers asked whether he had been up the evening before on an all-night assignment.

Upon examining him, I quickly noted that his unrested appearance was the result of drooping eyebrows. The before and after photographs below demonstrate the improvement in his condition accomplished by a surgical procedure known as brow-lifting surgery.

Heavy or low-set brows are a common cause of a tired or stern appearance in both men and women. When not taken to the extreme, repositioning drooping brows with surgery can result in a more alert and youthful appearance. However, it is important to take care when performing this procedure; overdoing the lift can result in an unnatural-appearing expression.

In the direct approach to a brow lift, incisions are generally placed in a natural wrinkle line and, once the healing process has run its course, are virtually imperceptible, as demonstrated in the marshal's photographs above.

In both men and women, drooping of the eyebrows is frequently one of the first signs of aging. This condition is often overlooked because most people are unaware of the problem and the degree of improvement its correction can provide.

A heavy eyebrow also causes the upper lids to drop or descend until, in the advanced stages, eyelid skin can touch or overlap the eyelashes. (See the previous photographs.) Prior to correction, patients often complain that their eyes appear to be getting smaller or more deeply set. Women note that eye makeup usually ends up high on the upper part of the lids a short while after it is applied.

Sagging eyebrows may be improved by a forehead lift (with incisions hidden at or within the hairline) or by excising skin in a wrinkle line above the drooping section of the brow. Both procedures lift the brow and surrounding tissues into a more youthful position, which—when performed in keeping with the recommendations set forth in this book— results in eyes that appear ten to fifteen years younger.

Following eyebrow-lifting surgery, there is often lessening of the deeper crow's feet found next to the outer corners of the eye. However, for the best result, those wrinkles might also require a skin-resurfacing procedure. In my experience, chemical peeling works best for this region of the face. Neuromodulators (such as Botox, Dysport, and Xeomin) can also provide temporary improvement in the crow's feet that occur when the muscles in that region are contracted.

The eyebrow lift will not correct excess skin or pouching caused by fat herniation at the inner corners of the upper lids, and it will not have any effect on lower-lid conditions. On the other hand, the procedure can be—and often is—effectively combined with surgery designed to improve problems in other regions of your face.

Most appearance-enhancement surgeons prefer to accomplish an eyebrow lift in conjunction with the temporal or forehead portion of a facelift, but in some cases, the procedure can be performed without any additional surgery or injectable therapies.

Some surgeons prefer to perform brow-lifting surgery through smaller incisions with the use of an endoscope, a lighted tube inserted beneath the skin of the brow and forehead. The downside of any brow-lifting procedure with incisions made behind the frontal hairline is that as the brows are lifted, so is the frontal hairline. Only by making corrective incisions at or below the frontal hairline can the hairline remain in a natural position.

When deep creases are present, the muscles that allow for forehead expressions might also be surgically interrupted. In the next chapter, we'll explore the cheek and neck portions of facial rejuvenation.

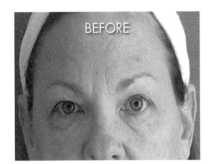

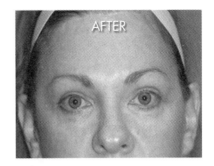

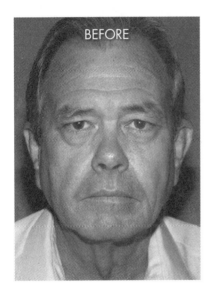

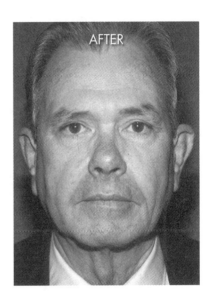

CHAPTER 20

The Facelift Operation

The Greek word for wrinkle is *rhytid*. The suffix *-ectomy* means "to remove"; thus, *rhytidectomy* is the medical term for the operation designed to lift, improve, or remove wrinkles caused by sagging tissues in the forehead, face, and neck.

The term "facelift" is often used to describe any renovation project, not necessarily one of a surgical nature. Sometimes the term is applied to renovating buildings, gardens, or vintage automobiles, airplanes, or boats. In uninformed medical circles, the term is also used incorrectly to describe a total facial rejuvenation, which includes eyelid surgery and perhaps skin resurfacing. While a muscle-suspension facelift and selective liposuction provide a large part of the foundation for a total rejuvenation process, other procedures I address in this book provide the finishing touches. By no means, however, does this mean that every patient who requests a facelift must agree to additional procedures. I remind you of the condition-specific approach to facial rejuvenation addressed previously. In that system, only the areas that need to be addressed at that particular time in a patient's life are addressed—and with the patient's consent.

The goal of any facelift operation is to reduce the sagging and wrinkling caused by ever-mounting loose skin. More advanced and long-lasting techniques also lift or reposition both the muscles and fatty tissues of the face and neck into the more youthful positions they once occupied, recreating the volume that once existed. An often overlooked fact of the rejuvenation process is that even once the drooping tissues of the face and neck are repositioned, the aging process continues. It is much like setting a clock to an earlier time or picking up an object and repositioning it farther back on a conveyor belt. Unless the clock or conveyor belt is stopped, the object continues to move ever closer to the position it once occupied. The same is true of the aging tissues in our bodies, including those in our faces, eyelids, and necks.

In my experience, when the drooping tissues of the face are repositioned into their more youthful states, underlying implants and fat injections are rarely indicated.

As described in previous chapters, unless the forehead portion of a facelift is performed, you will not obtain improvement in drooping brows. Nor does a facelift correct conditions of your upper or lower eyelids or the wrinkles or creases in your lips. Other procedures referenced earlier in this book (blepharoplasty, brow lifting, or skin resurfacing) are required to improve these conditions.

For decades, the facelift operation has been one of the most popular cosmetic operations performed in the head and neck regions of the human body. As medical advances and new technology increase the average life span, many people find that they look older than they feel, physically and mentally.

As the sociological mores of an ever-progressing society take shape, the stigma once associated with undergoing appearance-enhancing plastic surgery is rapidly disappearing. Men and women from all walks of life are giving themselves opportunities to look as healthy and youthful as they feel. The techniques I use—and in many instances have developed—are designed to restore your face to a naturally more youthful appearance.

As a potential consumer, it is important that you be aware that the facelift operation can be divided into three parts: the forehead or eyebrow lift (the upper third), the cheek lift (the middle third), and the neck lift (the lower third). The majority of people past the age of fifty seeking facial rejuvenation require all three components, but depending on your own conditions at the time of your consultation, you might require surgery in only one or two areas. An elite facial surgeon will advise you in your particular situation. Most people seeking neck lifts require some lifting of the cheeks in order to avoid puckering of the skin around their ears. You may or may not require a cheek lift or liposuction, but an elite surgeon will demonstrate the pros and cons of doing so. If the surgeon you consult does not suggest a cheek lift in addition to a neck lift, ask them to explain why or why not. As with any procedure, you are entitled to being duly advised.

Depending upon the time in your life when you consider age-reversing surgery, face-lifting surgery might be indicated to help you maintain a youthful face or to assist you in recapturing much of the youthful appearance that you had some ten to fifteen years previously.

In recent years, nonsurgical or minimally invasive surgical procedures have been promoted by the companies that manufacture various devices and machines. It is important for consumers and providers alike to keep in mind that an authentic facelift addresses drooping fatty tissue and muscles as well as sagging skin. The nonsurgical "facelifts" performed by an assembly-line manufactured machine are incapable of addressing the sagging fat and muscles of the face and neck. At the time of this writing, there is only one way to rejuvenate the deeper layers of an aging face: condition-specific and skillfully performed rejuvenating surgery that includes lifting and supporting the muscles and fat of the face with techniques that have stood the test of time.

If you are contemplating appearance-enhancing surgery, it is natural for you to want to know how much improvement you can expect and the duration of that improvement. In reality, the amount of improvement obtained with appearance-enhancing surgery depends upon a number of factors, not the least of which include the degree of wrinkling and sagging present, the quality of your skin, and the skills and experience of the specialist chosen to perform the procedures.

When the signs of aging are excessive, the postsurgical results can be dramatic, often allowing my patients to appear as much as fifteen to twenty years younger than their chronological ages. If the undesirable signs of aging are occurring prematurely and the recommended procedures are being performed in an attempt to *maintain* a youthful appearance, the improvement will obviously be more subtle. Friends might comment that you appear "less tired" and "look more alive, rested, and fresher." Some of my patients say that they are told they appear to have lost weight, because the heaviness along their jawline and in their neck was improved by a combination of liposuction and of lifting sagging muscles and skin into a more youthful position.

How Long Does a Facelift Last?

In reality, the results achieved through a facelift (or any surgical facial rejuvenation procedure) last forever in that the aged tissues removed at the time of surgery are permanently discarded. As previously mentioned, the skin and muscles beneath your drooping skin were surgically repositioned into their more youthful state. Even so, however, all the structures and tissues in your face and neck continue to age from their newly lifted positions. So, patients who have undergone facelifts can expect to see a gradual return of the conditions corrected with appearance-enhancement surgery as their aging process continues. To put it another way, any droops, sags, or wrinkles that appear following surgery are the result of the never-ending aging process, not an indication that aging tissues were not properly addressed at the time of your surgery.

Many patients who seek rejuvenation surgery are not informed of this truth, fail to grasp it, or fail to ask about it. Not until they begin to see a return of some of the ever-mounting signs of aging does their surgeon attempt to explain what is happening.

When I lecture to my appearance-enhancing colleagues at continuing medical education seminars, I remind them of a statement I coined some thirty years ago: "What we (physicians and surgeons) tell our patients prior to surgery or treatment falls under the category of 'informed consent.' The things we attempt to explain afterward are considered by our patients to be excuses."

As a more fully informed consumer, you are now equipped with knowledge and insight not possessed by too many of the women and men who blindly give over their faces, bodies, and futures to the ever-expanding appearance-enhancement industrial complex. This places you in a unique position. You can have a greater say in the process of becoming the person of your dreams.

In addition to providing my patients with a practice-specific consumer information book (*The Appearance Factor*), I display the following admonitions on the wall immediately facing them during their postoperative visits. In addition, I provide a prerecorded narrative to the patients with whom I consult. The recorded message addresses the postoperative course they should expect. I now also provide some of the same admonitions to you and to my appearance-enhancing colleagues around the world.

PATIENT REMINDERS
For Facial Surgery . . .

1. Don't try to evaluate the results too soon.
2. Healing times vary from one person to the other.
3. Swelling (and bruising) goes away.
4. Scars tend to improve with time.
5. Thick scars may be improved with cortisone treatments.
6. Tightness indicates swelling; don't pull against it.
7. Saggy-baggy tissues are a result of continued aging.
8. Loose skin seen after surgery was not left behind.
9. Protect peeled and dermabraded skin as you would a baby's skin.
10. Follow Instructions.

"Loose skin seen following surgery was not left behind" underscores the revelations I have shared in this and other chapters related to facelift and eyelid operations. I routinely inform my patients of the amount of loose skin that was removed at the time of their surgery and remind them of the information I provided prior to their surgery regarding how the healing process will play out. I remind them that the tightness and numbness in their cheeks and neck in the weeks following surgery is part of the healing process; that any elastic material (human skin included) that is stretched will loosen and sag over time; and that overly stretching the skin during surgery to compensate for the aging that will follow is what leaves so many plastic surgery patients with the overdone appearance that can—and should—be avoided.

How soon you might choose to have an appearance-enhancing surgeon address *new* signs of aging (those expected following your surgery) depends upon your personal and professional lifestyle management plan.

You will recall that, in earlier chapters, I described helping you become (and remain, for years to come) the person of your dreams as a partnership—an ongoing process that requires the best efforts of both of us.

If, prior to surgery, the wrinkling or sagging of facial and eyelid tissues was severe, it will obviously take years before the condition becomes equally noticeable. If, because of the self-induced conditions addressed in other chapters of this book, your own aging process is occurring more rapidly than usual, new wrinkling and sagging in the face and neck will also occur more rapidly. The fact that I and my fellow surgeons can address only conditions that *currently* exist and cannot bring to a halt the aging process is precisely why less extensive (and less expensive) "tuck-up" procedures are part of the lifelong appearance-enhancement master plan that I offer to my patients. However, the necessary foundation upwhich tuck-ups are based can be established only if the deeper structures (sagging muscles and fat) of your face are addressed in the first operation. If only a tuck was performed initially, a suspension facelift will be necessary.

When patients consult me after having undergone surgery with other surgeons, I recommend they obtain a copy of their operative report from their previous surgeon. Without that report, I am at a loss for what was or was not done by previously, making it more difficult (though not impossible) to plan the procedure I intend to perform.

So many age-reversing procedures are interrelated. I remind you that, as it relates to the face and neck, liposuction removes unwanted fat along the jawline and in the neck. In most cases, when combined with surgical tightening of your sagging muscles and skin, liposuction can improve your results by as much as 20–25 percent. If your face is simply "fat," it might be improved through liposuction and removing the associated sagging muscles and skin. However, due to the weight exerted on the skin of the face and neck, the results you achieve will be apparent for shorter periods of time. In such cases, and because youthful skin has better elasticity than aged skin, in keeping with my condition-specific approach to facial rejuvenation I might recommend only liposuction.

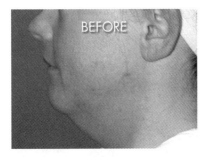 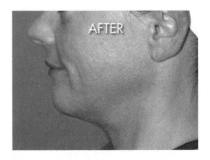

Liposuction alone was performed on this patient.

As an aside, the ability to intentionally stretch skin (via medical-grade expanders or serial excisions of scarred tissue or previously applied skin grafts) is a useful technique in reconstructive plastic surgery, especially when repairing defects created by cancer removal, excessive traumatic scarring, or birth-related abnormalities. These techniques take advantage of the fact that any skin placed under tension will stretch. The process is similar to how the skin of a woman's abdomen stretches during the last two trimesters of pregnancy as a result of the ever-expanding uterus and baby inside.

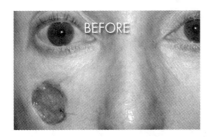 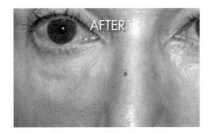

In some cases, the duration of time between a condition-specific facelift and an continuing-maintenance "tuck" can be as much as ten to fifteen years. Remember that the goal of age-reversing surgery is to create for you a face that is similar to the one you had some ten to fifteen years previously. However, if you wish to maintain the appearance of an ageless face, you may wish to return for minor tweaks and tucks before the proverbial conveyor belt of time reaches the ten- to fifteen-year mark.

Regardless of what you have read or been told, no operation or commercially available product currently known to man can predictably prevent aging. If so, I would be not only touting that product or procedure in this treatise but incorporating it into my everyday life and recommending it to my patients and family.

Here's what I hope you will remember: rejuvenation procedures and products are capable of addressing only the conditions present at any given time in your life. However, following a facelift—or any surgical rejuvenating procedure—you should never thereafter appear as old as you would had those procedures not been performed. This statement does not apply to temporary injectable therapies. Once the filler or neuromodulator has been absorbed or neutralized by your body, the natural state of aging that previously existed reappears.

In addition to the "conveyor belt of time" paradigm, I often use the "clock of life reset" example. Imagine a clock steadily ticking along. Then imagine the time registered on that same clock being set back ten to fifteen years. Then imagine the same clock continuing to tick along at the same pace as it did before the reset took place. With each passing second, the clock approaches the time it registered prior to being reset, until, ten to fifteen years in the future, it reaches that time. However, had that clock—the clock that registers the time of your life—not been reset with rejuvenating surgery, the physical signs of aging would be far more advanced than they might currently appear. This is why it is accurate to say that a well-conceived and skillfully performed facelift lasts for as long as you live. It is also accurate to say that any signs of aging you notice following a facelift are a result of the continuation of the aging process, not necessarily the result of a poorly performed surgical procedure—at least, not as long as the excess fatty tissues and the sagging of the muscles of the face and neck were properly addressed. This is why you should be assured that your surgeon plans to suspend sagging muscles and fat as well as skin.

I remind you of a point I emphasized earlier in this chapter: not all facelifts and skin-rejuvenation procedures and products are the same. In that regard, if you determine that you might be a candidate for appearance-enhancing procedures, consider giving yourself the knowledge and insight I offer in this book. You might also ask the following questions of the professional or professionals you choose to consult.

- "Am I asking the right questions?"
- "Am I consulting with the right providers of appearance- and health-enhancement procedures and products?"
- If either of the previous questions is not answered to your satisfaction, the follow-up question is: "Where else can I turn for the answers I seek?"

I'd like to believe that this book is the answer to the vast majority of your questions. I would hope that it provides guidance to those whose questions continue to linger. If you have further questions, I invite you to visit my website, McColloughPlasticSurgery.com. If you enter a question or concern, I will respond directly to you. Attaching a photograph of the condition about which you are concerned will expedite the eConsult process. Keep in mind that eConsult recommendations are preliminary in nature and are offered as a public service free of charge. The final recommendations will not be rendered until I have an opportunity to examine you in person. However, it is a way for you to obtain recommendations without having to visit a surgeon's office.

Assuming that you proceed with my recommendations, you can be assured that when newly acquired signs of aging become a concern, a variety of tuck-up procedures can be performed as often as you desire (within reason). I say "within reason" because I have patients in my practice who suffer from body dysmorphic syndrome (BDS) who would have surgery every year or sooner if I would agree to perform it. As a mind/body/spirit metaphysician, I see it as my responsibility to recommend against surgery when other measures are indicated. Additional thoughts on this theme are provided in a subsequent chapter.

You should view with skepticism any claims that some surgeons' facelift techniques last longer. The secret to longer-lasting results is whether the muscles underneath the sagging skin were properly suspended into a more youthful position and whether the sagging and ever-accumulating fatty tissues were adequately addressed. Particularly when done by inexperienced hands, dissecting far into the face and exposing the nerves that control facial movements (deep-plane face lifting) is fraught with problems and all manner of disappointments, as is overly stretching the skin of your face and neck in an attempt to have a tight postoperative appearance for a longer time.

The underlying foundation created by an initial condition-specific facial rejuvenation creates the desired situation for a future tuck-up. It is important to remember, however, that it is not necessary that you undergo additional cosmetic surgery. The tuck-up operation is simply an integral part of an ongoing rejuvenation maintenance program.

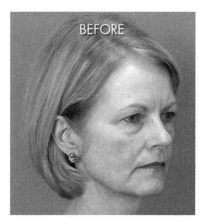 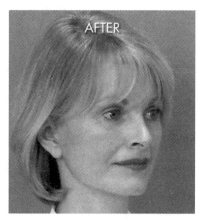

Early signs of aging corrected with a stage 3 facelift and eyelid surgery.

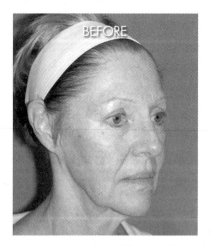 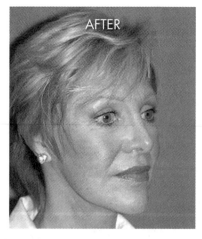

Stage 4 face lifting with eyelid and nasal rejuvenation surgery.

CHAPTER 21

The Rejuvenation Process:

What You Might Not Otherwise Be Told

Not every person seeking rehabilitation of the aging skin of their face and neck is an acceptable candidate for surgery. Those with known serious medical and psychological problems (including body dysmorphic syndrome) are usually excluded. Patients who are obese or who have a short, thick neck have little chance of a worthwhile and lasting result. This is why, in earlier sections of this book, I emphasize weight management as an integral part of life and appearance-enhancing therapies. The severe "turkey gobbler" deformity that occurs in the neck of some individuals can best be corrected by a direct excision of excess skin and fat from an incision placed in the midline of the neck under the chin. Finally, prospective patients who have unrealistic expectations—regardless of the procedures requested—are not candidates for appearance-enhancing procedures or products.

In keeping with the ways in which lifestyle contributes to the aging process—and to the procedures designed to address it—you should know that nicotine interferes with blood flow through the skin of the face, delays healing, and tends to increase the likelihood of postsurgical complications. I strongly recommend that prospective surgical candidates reveal to me whether they use any form of tobacco or smoking-cessation aids. Doing so will be in everyone's interest—theirs, mine, and that of those who care for and about them. Also know that based upon emerging evidence, vaping (the act of inhaling and exhaling an aerosol, often referred to as vapor, produced by an e-cigarette or similar device) is not proving to be a safe substitute for tobacco products.

Additional Facts about Facial Rejuvenation Surgery

When I perform facial rejuvenation procedures, surgical incisions are placed within the hair and around the ear so that they can be camouflaged by the adjacent hair or by the natural creases and folds of the ears. On rare occasions, there might be thinning of the hair around the incision line. If this phenomenon should occur, the area can be addressed by a minor touch-up procedure. However, the techniques I use are designed to protect and preserve hair and to minimize scarring.

If a temporal or forehead lift is performed, the hairline might be altered. However, I choose to use techniques that eliminate or minimize hairline alterations. In short, the operation is customized to fit the needs and desires of each patient seeking facial enhancement.

Reliable Skin Rejuvenation:
Off with the Old, On with the New

When considering total facial rejuvenation, smoother, wrinkle-free skin is a goal sought by my patients and by me. To confuse the matter, segments of the commercial cosmetic industry offer a plethora of products and procedures that unfortunately promote unrealistic expectations in some cases. In a previous chapter, I stressed that superficial treatments (level 1 procedures—the kinds that are offered in the Skin Center and Total Health Spa at the McCollough Institute) *polish* the top layers of the skin, leaving unaddressed the underlying conditions of aging in the deeper layers. These level 1 procedures, such as superficial peels and microdermabrasion, are incapable of correcting deeper wrinkles and addressing dreaded precancerous conditions. Treatments that penetrate more deeply (levels 2 and 3 procedures) generally take two to three weeks to heal and not only remove sun-damaged and wrinkled skin but actually create the new collagen and elastic tissues below the surface that less invasive procedures only promise

To help clear up the plethora of confusion around skin-rejuvenation procedures, I developed a previously mentioned classification that accurately describes the extent to which facial skin should be (and can be) safely exfoliated, a term that describes the removal of various layers of your skin from the surface down. As I am doing here, I stress to my patients that the end result of any exfoliating product or procedure is directly proportional to the depth (or penetration) of the treatment, meaning that although healing takes longer, more deeply penetrating treatments (levels 2 and 3) tend to yield better and longer-lasting results. Remember, when a provider talks about a procedure having no downtime, in reality they are telling you that no long-term results should be expected. Unless the skin-resurfacing procedure takes at least two weeks to heal, you cannot expect it to achieve the results that you might have been promised.

The microscopically thin outermost layer of skin (the stratum corneum of the epidermis) can clearly be removed with exfoliating cosmetics that contain glycolic, salicylic, or retinoic acid (Retin-A), or with those that contain some related acid. These can be applied at home or in a medical skin-enhancement center. I remind you that level 1 products and procedures tend to polish your skin, much in the same way that furniture polish makes old furniture shine, but only for a short while.

Other ways to remove superficial layers of skin and constrict dilated blood vessels below include IPL (intense pulse light), lasers, microdermabrasion, or stronger concentrations of the acid preparations mentioned above. These procedures are often available in *medical* spa settings—i.e., those that are owned and operated by physicians.

The crucial fact to remember is that none of the aforementioned level 1 treatments penetrate into the deeper layers of the skin. Because they do not, they are unable to reverse advanced sun damage, blemishes, or wrinkles. To have any long-lasting effect on these unwanted conditions, a skin-enhancement treatment must extend into the dermis (the deeper layers) and take a minimum of two weeks to heal. I urge you to keep this fact in mind as you seek skin-enhancement procedures and therapies. If you do, you will save yourself money and frustration in the years ahead.

Even if the treatment to which you agree does extend to the dermal layer, it is important to keep in mind that methods of removing or exfoliating skin are, more often than not, overexaggerated and overcommercialized. The end result of an appearance-enhancing treatment depends upon in whose hands the technology is placed. Like appearance-enhancing surgery, skin care is both an art and science. It cannot be learned in a weekend or by sitting in an audience at a medical convention.

Whether the doctor with whom you choose to consult uses lasers, dermabrasion, chemical peeling, or a combination of all three modalities, you should be told up front that the depth of penetration into your skin, not the type of technology used to initiate the rejuvenation process, determines the success or failure of any treatment alternative.

As with other remedies I recommend in this book, when considering a resurfacing procedure, the first step is to undergo a scientific skin analysis. Doing so determines the current health—or lack thereof—of your skin within each region of your face and body. Skin thickness, solar damage, acne scarring, or wrinkling might differ on different parts of the same face or body. Therefore, the treatment required for each area should be adjusted to the conditions identified in each region of your face or body by a trained skin-care professional.

The first—and often the most crucial step—in maintaining or enhancing the appearance of your skin is to determine which areas require treatment and which areas should be left undisturbed, at least for the time being. For example, as a well-advised patient, you might choose to treat the lines around your upper and lower lip or the wrinkles around your eyes but leave other areas of your face and body alone. In other cases, it might be best to resurface the entire face as well as your hands and forearms. By treating those areas at the right time in your aging process, your newly resurfaced skin will be more likely to blend in with the adjacent areas. An experienced appearance-enhancement surgeon can explain the various aesthetic units (regions) of your face and body and then recommend the most appropriate treatment for each area.

The next chapter delves more deeply into the art and science of rejuvenating skin-resurfacing procedures.

CHAPTER 22

The Rest of the Skin-Rejuvenation Story

The late iconic actor and radio personality Paul Harvey was famous for following up on the news of the day with what he called "the rest of the story." In keeping with Mr. Harvey's attempt to go beyond any abbreviated version of the facts, I offer the following.

The procedures I describe in this chapter are often labeled "nonsurgical facelifts." Although they are not a replacement for surgical tightening of facial muscles and removal of excess skin, they do create *some* enhancement in terms of reversing the aging process. I emphasize the word *some*.

In the 1980s, I conducted a facial rejuvenation convention in Birmingham. In addition to lectures, I included live surgery so that the attendees could see the surgery taking place in real time. Although the patient whose photographs are included below might have benefitted from a face and neck lift, her doctor had prescribed blood-thinning medications (anticoagulants) for a looming cardiovascular condition and recommended she not discontinue them, not even for a few days. As an alternative to a facelift, I recommended a level 3 chemical peel. The procedure not only corrected this patient's wrinkling but delivered on the promises she'd been made by producing new collagen and elastin in the dermal regions of the skin of her face that lifted the skin in her neck as well. Seeing the results she obtained, it is easy to understand why level 3 chemical peels are often referred to as nonsurgical facelifts.

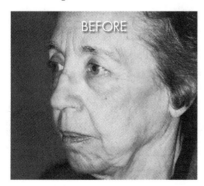 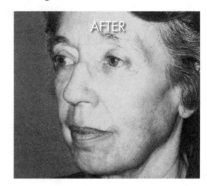

Creative, profit-driven, trademarked ways to apply peeling solutions do not change the fact that the appropriate mixture of chemicals causes a separation of the upper layer of skin, which peels or sheds within a few days much like a deeper sunburn would.

Clearly, superficial layers of skin can be removed by a variety of methods of skin resurfacing, including chemical peeling, dermabrasion, and laser resurfacing. Each technique seems to have some unique qualities—and limitations. My experience is that wrinkles are best corrected with chemical peeling and acne scars are best improved with dermabrasion. While I have not found lasers to be as effective as peeling and dermabrasion for these conditions, in experienced hands, lasers can create some degree of improvement. An experienced surgeon can explain which procedures might be the most advantageous in your case.

Throughout this book, I have referred to different levels of skin resurfacing. Until I developed the system that I use for my patients, these levels were known as "superficial, medium, and deep." Something about the word "deep" made many of my patients uncomfortable. So I decided to come up with a different method for referring to the depth of the treatment I recommended. My new classification not only is more anatomically descriptive but seems to be more acceptable to my patients. See whether you agree.

Level 1: This level of treatment is often offered by nonsurgeons, frequently in a spa setting. Patients are able to return to work, home, or play immediately. Little or no healing time is required. Level 1 treatments tend to polish the skin for a few weeks but create essentially no long-term benefits.

Level 2: These procedures are generally offered by facial plastic surgeons and dermatologists. More layers (levels) of damaged and wrinkled skin are removed with these deeper treatments to the upper dermis. Healing time generally requires about two weeks. Level 2 procedures are generally recommended for patients younger than fifty years old or those with minimal to moderate sun damage and wrinkling.

Level 3: These procedures should be performed by facial plastic surgeons or surgically oriented dermatologists. Level 3 resurfacing procedures penetrate into the deeper dermis, where collagen and elastic fibers are produced; therefore, they are the most effective methods of removing severely sun-damaged and precancerous skin, as well as skin that contains deeper pigmentation or wrinkles. Healing time is longer—generally three weeks; however, the results are longer lasting and dramatic.

Different parts of your face (or, in some cases, your body) generally require differing levels or depths of treatment. For example, the thin skin of your eyelids might not tolerate the same level of treatment that the thicker skin of your forehead, nose, lips, and chin might require. An experienced surgeon will know how to vary the depth of the treatment to meet your specific needs.

With any of these methods, outer layers of sun-damaged, aged, wrinkled, or scarred skin are removed. However, only with level 2 and 3 procedures are new collagen and elastic fibers produced in the deeper layers of skin—more so in level 3 treatments than level 2. Only when the dermal layers deeper in the skin are challenged do new collagen and elastin fibers replace the old, and only then does tightening of the skin occur. However, it does not occur to the extent that can be accomplished with surgical suspension and removal through conventional face-lifting and eyelid-lifting techniques.

The superficial (level 1) peels that are offered by many spas and nonsurgical offices and clinics (including mine) generally do not produce long-term improvement in the quality and texture of the skin. However, they might be useful as skin-polishing adjuncts *after* level 2 and 3 methods have been performed.

The Truth about Wrinkles

Neither a facelift, eyelid surgery (blepharoplasty), nor a brow lift will totally remove the wrinkles of weather-beaten skin, the horizontal creases of the forehead, the crow's feet around the outer corners of the eyes, or the vertical wrinkles of the upper and lower lips. Remember, surgery is designed to improve sags and bulges, whereas the skin-resurfacing procedures I address in this book are designed to improve wrinkles.

Level 2 and especially level 3 resurfacing procedures usually cause the skin to have a more youthful fullness—a rewarding and frequently dramatic change that has been described as being like peaches instead of prunes.

Along with topically applied bleaching agents, the more invasive skin-resurfacing procedures (peeling or dermabrasion) might improve the diffuse, patchy pigmentation that sometimes accompanies or follows pregnancy or chronic skin irritations, regardless of the underlying cause. However, as I addressed earlier, the best treatment of any condition lies in identifying the underlying cause as well as the conditions left in the cause's wake.

Skin-bleaching procedures and products can also improve the troublesome dark circles that some people experience under their eyes—assuming, that is, that the circles are caused by darkly pigmented skin rather than shadowing created by bulging fat.

Skin resurfacing can be performed as an isolated procedure—around the lips, for example, around the eyes, or over your entire face. It can also be used as an indispensable adjunct to face lifting and eyelid plastic surgery in a comprehensive facial rejuvenation program. Before the turn of the twenty-first century, I was taught to wait three to six months before resurfacing areas in which skin had been tightened with surgery; however, in recent years, I have been performing level 2 skin resurfacing (chemical peeling and/or dermabrasion) at the same time as face lifting and blepharoplasty. Because the technique I use during face lifting and blepharoplasty preserves much of the blood supply to the flaps, resurfacing can be combined with other rejuvenating procedures.

Some skin types respond more favorably to skin-resurfacing procedures than others. Fair complexions tend to have less posttreatment discoloration than dark ones; however, over my career, I have learned that when it comes to the human condition, the only absolute is this: imponderables can never be discarded. I learned this irrefutable principle directly from famed heart surgeon Dr. John Kirklin. When it comes to skin resurfacing, skin that is thick, tough, more deeply etched, or oily might require a two-stage approach for the best results—that is, a second peel or touch up of several areas at a later time. As with painting any roughly textured surface, an additional coat of resurfacing might be beneficial.

Except in extreme cases (such as the patient discussed at the beginning of this chapter), resurfacing alone is not generally indicated for treatment of sagging tissues. Although your new skin will have better elasticity following skin resurfacing, sagging tissues beneath your skin will be more reliably improved with surgical suspension. Even so, during my forty-six-year career as a facial plastic surgeon, I have observed additional tightening in the skin in many patients after levels 2 and 3 resurfacing, to such an extent that additional surgery was not indicated.

You should also know that taking female hormones or birth control pills after a resurfacing procedure before all pink discoloration has subsided might lead to changes in your skin's color. Patients who feel they must take hormones usually do so without incurring any problems. Also, today bleaching agents are effective in treating darkly pigmented areas, should they occur.

Following skin resurfacing, postoperative care is extremely important to obtain the best result possible. Your newly resurfaced skin will have many of the characteristics of the skin of a newborn baby. It will take time for it to toughen and be able to tolerate direct sun, wind exposure, salt air, and certain skin-care products. Because it is new skin, the texture and color will be somewhat different from skin that was not resurfaced. It might look more like the skin on your body that has never been exposed to sunlight. Makeup can generally camouflage any contrasts in color between your new and untreated skin. Superficial (levels 1 and 2) resurfacing procedures can be used in areas that cannot tolerate level 3 procedures, such as the neck, décolletage, arms, and hands.

You should also know that resurfacing procedures will not reduce the size of pores. A pore is the opening of an oil gland or hair follicle at the skin's surface. Attempts to reduce its size may lead to the development of a pimple. The exceptions are deep pores associated with rhinophyma, a skin condition that produces thick, irregular skin on the nose. The deep and wide pores in these patients may be improved with dermabrasion or laser therapy.

Resurfacing procedures can often produce a dramatic improvement in the texture of the skin of the face. When it comes to helping create fresher, more youthful skin, the resurfacing procedures discussed here offer the best—and most reliable—treatments available. Level 2 or 3 skin resurfacing is certainly not indicated for every patient, however, and reputable surgeons will give you their opinion as to whether they feel you are a candidate for these procedures.

Ongoing professional care of your new skin is important to help you maintain the results that have been accomplished with resurfacing. With that thought in mind, if you are considering a skin-resurfacing procedure, you should inform your appearance-enhancement surgeon if you have taken Accutane. While Accutane can often work wonders in treating cystic acne, it delays healing from resurfacing procedures and can result in serious complications. I recommend that patients wait at least a year after discontinuing Accutane before undergoing anything more than a level 1 resurfacing procedure.

Injectable Wrinkle Therapy: Botox, Fillers, and Fat

In recent years, there has been an explosion in the use of many nonsurgical techniques and devices that claim to rejuvenate an aging face. It is my conviction—and the conviction of most elite appearance-enhancement professionals—that more dramatic, decisive, and favorable improvements are accomplished when the appropriate time-honored surgical techniques discussed in this book are thoughtfully and skillfully applied.

In some patients, however, neuromodulators (Botox, Dysport, or Xeomin), fat, and fillers can be used to treat early unfavorable facial changes. Neuromodulators (muscle paralyzing agents) produce the desired effect by temporarily paralyzing specific muscles of facial expression—the ones that cause wrinkling when called into action.

During the past two decades, neuromodulator injections have gained widespread popularity. They can be used for a variety of facial issues, including lessening crow's feet and wrinkles of the forehead and the chin caused by contracting the muscles in those regions. This effect is different from the results accomplished with resurfacing, which improves the wrinkles present *at rest*. This is a fact that must be incorporated into any total facial rejuvenation plan, especially *yours!*

However, when addressing the wrinkles in your face, the best results are generally obtained by using a combination of neuromodulators and resurfacing. Neuromodulators may also be injected to improve some of the spasms and asymmetry that patients with facial paralysis, Bell's palsy, and blepharospasm experience. It should be noted that neuromodulator results are not permanent and will need to be repeated. You should also know that the time between treatments varies from one person to the other. Your body may metabolize muscle-paralyzing agents faster than other patients' bodies and therefore require more frequent treatments. If so, you should ask your injection professional about alternative neuromodulator products.

The next three chapters delve more deeply into the specific skin-resurfacing procedures I have addressed in this and other chapters. When you read them, you will know as much as many of the professionals that you might consult. As such, you are likely to receive the treatments and care you require.

As I wrote the paragraph above, the saying "forewarned is forearmed" came to mind. While receiving the best care and advice on your way to becoming the person of your dreams should not be a contest of wills, it is certainly a contest of priorities—yours and those of the appearance- and health-enhancement professionals you choose to be on your team. When choosing the members of that team, do not ignore this other snippet of wisdom: "If all one has is a hammer, everything begins to look like a nail." Your wrinkled, aging skin should never be looked upon as a nail.

CHAPTER 23

Chemical Peeling:

A Time-Tested Elixir for Aging Skin

In the broadest sense, an "elixir" is defined as something "miraculous, magical, and maybe a little mysterious . . . a sweet substance or solution that cures the problem at hand."[8] With linguistic roots in the long-ago alchemists' search for the philosopher's stone, the word adds an element of fantasy to spice up anything, even a remedy for the common cold. The mythic Fountain of Youth is certainly an elixir, but it can also refer to a real liquid, concept, or plan.

The "elixir" known as a Baker-Gordon chemical peel (also known as chemexfoliation) involves the careful application of a scientifically formulated solution to the skin that causes the top layer to predictably separate the undesirable layers from the regenerative ones over the ensuing days. The peeling process takes away the sun-damaged and wrinkled layers and creates a process in the remaining layers that regenerates the more desirable anatomy that existed prior to the patient's prolonged exposure to the damaging effects of the sun, overwhelming stress, or the unrelenting aging process. But a fact that you must remember is this: chemical peels differ in their ingredients and effects on your skin.

A level 2 or 3 peel is much like having been sunburned or having any heat-related blister. The top layer of skin begins to peel away over a four- to five-day period, revealing the fresh new deep-pink layer underneath. In contrast, a level 2 or 3 dermabrasion or laser treatment removes the unhealthy layers of the skin immediately.

---

8. Vocabulary.com, s.v. "elixir," accessed September 30, 2019, https://www.vocabulary.com/dictionary/elixir.

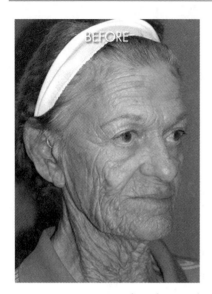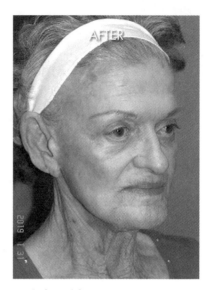

Level 3 chemical peeling with face lifting.

Regardless of the treatment modality, in most cases mineral powder makeup can be used to cover any pinkness that remains two or three weeks following treatment. However, because—in my experience—chemical peels provide the most effective treatment of facial wrinkles, healing often lags a few days behind dermabrasion and laser treatments. Most patients who undergo a level 2 or 3 skin-resurfacing procedure may return to work or go out socially within two to three weeks of treatment. When instructions and precautions are stringently adhered to, the deep-pink color of your newly resurfaced skin will slowly subside over the following six to eight weeks.

Posttreatment Limitations and Restrictions

The primary restriction after level 3 peeling is avoiding irritants or prolonged exposure to sunlight (as when sunbathing, fishing, golfing, etc.) for three to six months. Your "new" skin, like when you were a newborn baby, must build up a tolerance to the elements and noxious substances; otherwise, you could develop pigmentation issues and skin irritation in the treated areas. Since the advent of sunscreen products, and with the use of large-brimmed hats, these restrictions can sometimes be loosened. With the possible consequences looming, however, you should ask about any activity, product, or substance you question.

In my practice, I remind my patients about the long-term restrictions of activities following a peel or dermabrasion. Many of them have heard that once they have had a peel, dermabrasion, or laser procedure, they can never go out in the sun again. This, too, has not been my experience.

Although it is important to avoid sun exposure and to use sunscreen products during the first six to nine months, ordinary sun exposure after that is allowed. As was the case in the earliest weeks of your life, it simply takes time for your new skin to build up a natural resistance to sun and wind.

CHAPTER 24

Dermabrasion:

Another Skin-Resurfacing Technique

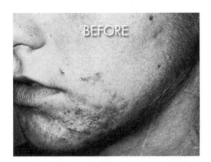 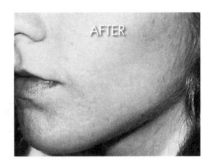

Cystic acne and scarring treated with dermabrasion.

When cystic acne does not respond to medical treatment, a level 3 therapeutic dermabrasion can often improve both the appearance and the medical problems in the affected areas. The procedure can be repeated, if necessary, within several months. Although I do not contend that dermabrasion is a treatment for every case of acne, many patients have received some improvement following this procedure. Acne is generally a medical condition, not a surgical one; therefore, its treatment should be supervised by the patient's dermatologist or a facial surgeon trained in Accutane therapy.

To emphasize this point, I share with you the story of a patient who was referred to me in the 1980s by the dermatology department at UAB's medical center. She had been treated with all therapies available at the time but continued to suffer with cystic acne and the related scarring.

I performed a level 3 therapeutic dermabrasion on this young woman. The results demonstrated in the photographs below show not only that there was an improvement in the appearance of her skin but that the intractable cystic acne from which she suffered disappeared, affirming my premise that the appearance and health of your skin are more closely related than many of my colleagues—and many insurance companies—are willing to accept.

The case I shared above underscores the fact that for patients whose skin exhibits an irregular or uneven texture from acne scarring or from previous injuries, a level 2 or 3 dermabrasion is often the right treatment. Another unappreciated fact is that dermabrasion is also a helpful adjunct to laser resurfacing when treating wrinkled, sun-damaged, or deeply pigmented areas of skin. This is especially true of fractioned laser therapy because it addresses only a fraction of the area treated. The lasered skin in the treated areas is usually wiped away with a surgical gauze pad. A better alternative is dermabrasion of the lasered areas. Doing so not only removes the lasered debris but provides a deeper level of treatment—and, therefore, a better posttreatment result,

Depending upon the settings that the operator chooses, somewhere between a third and half of the treated area might be skipped over by the fractioned laser beam. This is why healing time is reduced with fraction-ated therapies; a significant portion of the area is left untreated.

Like chemical peeling, dermabrasion addresses the entire area and is similar to sanding scratches of various depths from a wooden table in that the elevated areas around the depressions are abraded down closer to the depth of the defects.

In the vast majority of cases, a level 2 or 3 dermabrasion diminishes the high-low junctions which are responsible for casting shadows when light strikes the face from an angle, leaving the skin somewhat smoother and tighter than before. When the texture of the facial skin is irregular from excessive or deep scarring, a second treatment might be required six to twelve months after the initial treatment.

The drawings below represent an area of skin that might contain scars and defects of different widths, depths, and configurations.

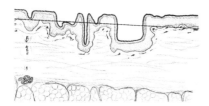 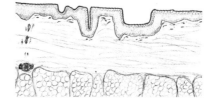

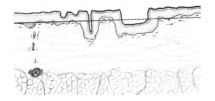 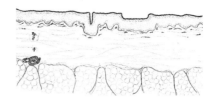

As the drawings demonstrate, the more superficial skin defects might be completely removed by dermabrasion. Those that are moderately deep might be improved but not removed, and some of the deeper or "icepick-type" scars might not be improved at all.

As the drawings indicate, in some cases, a second dermabrasion within six to twelve months can provide additional improvement to moderately deep scars. In rare circumstances, dermabrasion can be done a third time, but there is a limit. Prior to surgery, it is difficult to predict the degree of improvement and how *your* skin will respond to the treatment. However, the more experienced the surgeon, the better equipped they will be to predict the surgical outcome.

Skin pores are the surface openings of the oil glands. Neither dermabrasion, laser, nor a chemical peel can safely alter them.

Now that you have been forewarned with the facts provided in this chapter and the previous one, let's take an equally critical look at laser-assisted skin resurfacing.

CHAPTER 25

Laser-Assisted Skin Rejuvenation

Not all lasers are the same; nor are all operators of lasers. Lasers and their operators come in a variety of forms. Regardless of its manufacturer, a laser is no more than an instrument in the hands of its operator. As a duly informed consumer, you must realize that different lasers are designed to address different conditions. Contrary to popular belief, a laser is not the long-sought "magic wand" of mythological lore.

By concentrating a beam of light down to a pinpoint, some lasers vaporize the outer layers of sun-damaged or aging skin. By increasing the power settings, some can also pass through the outer layers of the skin and destroy deeper birthmarks (such as port-wine stains) or tiny blood vessels (spider veins). Others can intentionally damage the roots of hair (follicles) so that they are less likely to produce unwanted hair.

In short, lasers—like many of the therapies discussed in this book—are tools made available to a cross section of operators with varying degrees of training and expertise by commercially driven manufacturers. As is the case with most tools, brushes, and sculpting technologies, there is an art to using lasers. In order to obtain the maximum benefit, *experience* is the common denominator required to achieve the desired result.

What the average consumer does not know is that a physician can simply attend a convention and purchase a laser. A few weeks later, the laser will be delivered to the doctor, and following a two-hour training session, the doctor or one of his assistants can be performing laser-assisted procedures on trusting patients.

This is why I recommend throughout this book that, as a consumer, you need to ask the hard questions, beginning with, "How long have you been performing the procedure you are recommending for me?" Then you should follow up with, "Can you show me pre- and posttreatment images of patients you have personally treated?"

As a general rule, you do not want to be part of an experimental process. You should insist that the providers to whom you give your trust are experienced in performing the procedures they recommend to you.

Lasers, like any instrument, tool, or technology, must be used for the right reasons. The previous reference about hammers and nails applies to lasers. If a surgeon has a laser, they are apt to use it even when equally effective nonlaser options are available. The right time to use a laser is when laser technology is superior to other techniques. For some conditions, lasers exceed other forms of treatment. For others, chemical peeling and dermabrasion have proven more effective. The following paragraphs elaborate on this point.

Laser-Assisted Hair Removal

Unwanted hair on various parts of the body haunts both men and women. Fortunately, some lasers can assist in minimizing or eliminating much of this problem. Laser therapy can remove existing hair; however, individual hairs that are just developing and have not yet come through the skin might require future treatment.

The most effective hair-reduction treatment protocols usually take three to six treatments. Sessions are scheduled approximately six weeks apart. After these treatments, most patients will have no growth of hair in the treated areas for a period of time that can vary from months to years. Why the longevity of the treatments differs has not yet been determined; however, ongoing science might soon provide answers.

In reality, laser hair removal should be referred to as hair *reduction*, because no matter what form of laser therapy is used, a small percentage of hair will always grow back. Patients who experience regrowth of hair, however, usually notice a finer, less dense population in the treated areas. That's where electrolysis enters the picture. Shocking the roots of each hair with low-voltage electricity is the most reliable way to permanently eliminate it. As with the other therapies addressed in this book, electrolysis should be performed only by professionals who possess the training and experience necessary to avoid complications and produce acceptable results.

A physician can apply or inject anesthetic agents into the treated areas to make laser-assisted hair removal and electrolysis less painful. In addition, scarring is much less apt to occur with laser hair removal than when electrolysis is performed by a poorly trained and less-experienced aesthetician. Laser-assisted removal of unwanted facial hair is more effective on dark hairs. The fine, light-colored hairs on your face or arms do not respond as well to laser therapy.

The advantage of laser hair reduction is that it is a safe, cost-effective method with few side effects. In addition, it is the most effective semi-permanent method of hair reduction approved by the FDA. As with any other treatment, outcomes vary; however, having a physician perform or oversee the treatment is of extreme importance. It is the best way to minimize discomfort, achieve the maximum beneficial outcome, and reduce the possibility of adverse effects or complications.

Dilated Blood Vessels, Rosacea, and Pigmented Spots

After years of unprotected sun exposure, your skin will lose its smooth, uniform, youthful appearance. If you doubt the preceding statement, you need only examine your own skin on parts of your body that are not ordinarily exposed to the sun, such as the buttocks and your pubic areas. Keep in mind that when we are born, the skin on every part of our bodies is soft, smooth, and free of age spots. It is what you choose to do—or not to do—that determines how rapidly and severely your skin will age.

Certain chronic skin conditions (such as rosacea) can also cause damage to the collagen and elastic fibers of the dermal layers. Preventative maintenance and rejuvenation of your skin's collagen and elastic fibers can help maintain a youthful appearance. Skin conditions that are reliably improved by laser therapy include benign vascular lesions (telangiectasia, rosacea, flushing, and hemangiomas), sunspots, photoaging, different colorations in your skin, fine wrinkles, the large pores of rhinophyma, and loss of tone and elasticity.

The photographs below demonstrate the kind of improvement that can be obtained with laser therapy on aging hands.

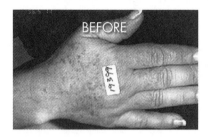
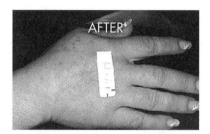

Leg Veins

Different types of lasers, offered by different manufacturers and distributors, have been used in the past three decades to address various kinds of vascular lesions, dilated veins, and capillaries. Also included in these troublesome defects within and below your skin are varicose veins of different sizes and depths. Superficial vascular problems include small spider veins and larger varicose veins. Traditionally sclerotherapy (injections of a concentrated salt solution) and surgical intervention with stripping were once the main methods of treatment for patients with these problems. Today, however, lasers are being used to treat spider and varicose veins in the legs, ankles, and feet.

Some of the advantages of laser-assisted therapies as compared to traditional ones include a lower rate of side effects, a shorter healing time, and the absence of compression therapy after treatment.

Acne Therapy

Acne is a condition that affects approximately 80 percent of the human population. Usually, the condition results from the obstruction, inflammation, and infection of the oil glands of the skin. Acne normally appears during the adolescent years as hormonal changes cause the body's oil glands to become occluded. However, it can occur in adults as well, especially during women's menopausal years.

Different modalities of medical treatments for acne have been tried, including topical or systemic antibiotics, Accutane therapy, and hundreds of over-the-counter remedies. Unfortunately, many patients fail to respond to them. Now, there is an effective way to treat acne with few or no side effects: lasers and related light-therapy technology. These involve minimal pain, no downtime, and no systemic drug treatments.

Intense pulse light (IPL) treatments for acne may take only fifteen minutes. A minimum of eight treatments in a period of four weeks is the recommended interval of therapy. In severe cases, it might be necessary for a facial plastic surgeon to work with a dermatologist in order to provide the maximum degree of improvement.

The next chapter addresses ways that you might avoid needing some of the skin-resurfacing procedures I have discussed so far.

CHAPTER 26

Why Caring for Your Skin Helps Take Care of You

A few years ago, my wife's cousin consulted with me about the condition of the skin of her face. She shared with me that when she and my wife were teenagers, they would lie on the beach after having applied baby oil and iodine to their skin, soaking up the sun's rays from late morning until midafternoon.

The photographs below demonstrate the cumulative effects of unprotected sun exposure. Clearly, iodine and baby oil are not intended to protect the skin from the sun's harmful rays. On the contrary, this combination of products enhances their penetration. With a level 3 chemical peel, I was able to reverse much of the damage.

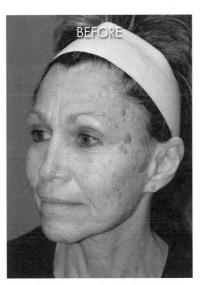 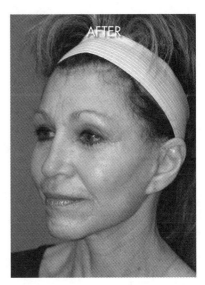

Fortunately, my wife's cousin did not develop skin cancer; however, the condition of her skin following intensive sun exposure should serve as a warning to young people to protect their own skin.

Did you know that your skin is the largest organ of your body and deserves as much attention as any other organ? It and its integumental extensions (hair and nails) are more than a body suit or an elastic covering for your internal organs. In addition to its role as a protective barrier to bacteria and other harmful organisms, your skin helps your body maintain a steady temperature and body-fluid level. Vitamin D (needed to keep bones strong) is also produced when sunlight comes into contact with your skin. Brittle bones have life-threatening implications. Years of abuse along with unprotected exposure to sun, wind, cold, and ultraviolet light cause the collagen and elastic fibers of your skin to break down and the lubricating and nutritional fluid elements between them to become sparse, leading to the development of dryness and wrinkles. Sun and wind exposure also cause abnormal cells to develop, leading to skin cancer and pigmented, splotchy blemishes. In keeping with choice-based health and beauty, nicotine and excessive alcohol intake can deplete your skin of essential nutrients and lead to premature aging.

Hormonal imbalances and improper cleansing can lead to acne and other chronic infections, which can cause scarring. Certain conditions of the nails of the hands and feet suggest the presence of a fungus (*Candida*) that can also set up house in other parts of the body.

The previous photographs demonstrate the kind of skin damage that can occur with years of excessive and unprotected sun exposure. Note the wrinkles and precancerous spots as well. These conditions were treated with a chemical peel, as described previously.

Finally, loss or brittleness of hair can be a sign of imbalance in the body's hormones, vitamins, or minerals. If your or those you care for have concerns about any of these issues, consultation with a physician is recommended.

A trained skin-care specialist working in harmony with a physician can help restore your skin to a more youthful level through rejuvenating therapy. They can also recommend treatments designed to keep your skin looking healthier for years to come. In addition, quality products—such as those offered by elite medical spas—can lubricate and protect your skin from some of the harmful environmental factors I described above. In some cases, products applied topically to your skin can help diminish discolored spots and regions.

The Hormone Factor

Hormone imbalances are another treatable cause of undesirable changes in your skin. This includes low thyroid levels (hypothyroidism). This condition causes your skin to become dry in some regions and puffy in others. Elevated thyroid levels (hyperthyroidism) can cause the skin to become thin and velvety smooth. Scientific testing of saliva and blood can determine whether your hormones, minerals, and vitamins are out of balance. Do not forget that hormone imbalances occur in men as well as in women.

Biocompatible hormone-replacement therapy can be initiated in both men and women, often restoring the body and mind to more youthful states of vitality. Once again, note that I use the term *biocompatible* rather than *bioidentical*. No nonhuman hormone substitute is exactly like the hormone of a human being; however, naturally occurring compounds found in yams and those manufactured in laboratories are similar and can be compatible with those ordinarily produced by our bodies. With advanced testing, other hormones not related to menopause or andropause can—and should—be scientifically measured. It is the most assured way to determine your holistic state of health.

In addition to the visible changes in the skin and body associated with thyroid imbalances, deficiencies or excesses of thyroid hormones and cortisone can produce conditions that cause a person to feel unwell. In some cases, severe imbalances can cause profound alterations in your appearance or become life threatening. Low levels of these hormones can cause you to feel tired and listless. High levels will cause you to feel overly stimulated and lead to aggressive behavior.

Skilled skin-care and holistic professionals can provide more information on these chemical and hormone imbalances and can work with your doctor to recommend the most appropriate doses and combinations of replacement therapy.

Professional Skin Care: Services and Products

Regardless of what you might have been told, human skin cannot be categorized into only four or five types. Because every individual in the world (other than identical twins) has a different genetic makeup, there are as many skin types as there are people.

Some products and technologies that claim to produce results in the deeper layers of your skin and underlying tissues are physically and chemically incapable of penetrating into the tissues they claim to rejuvenate. Because of this, it is impossible for them to achieve advertised objectives. Unless the deeper level of aging skin (the reticular dermis) is subjected to a controlled traumatic event (such as chemical peeling, dermabrasion, laser, radiofrequency, or microneedling), the treatment will not produce new, healthy collagen, fibrin, and elastin—the measurable building blocks associated with healthy, youthful-appearing skin.

When considering whether you should undergo the latest miracle treatment, the first question you should ask is this: Does the claim made by the promoter make scientific sense? Like all remedies, skin-care products and nutritional supplements ought to withstand the tests of scientific validity and professional oversight. "If it sounds too good to be true, it usually is too good to be true" is a good rule to follow.

For best results, skin-care and cosmetic products should be recommended only following a scientific skin analysis performed by a professional trained and experienced in the Rejuvenology sciences. In keeping with my prior advice about how one size *does not* fit all, skin-care products should be selected based on the diagnosis of a skin specialist, as well as on the product's effectiveness. My own research and experience indicate that no one company provides products that address the conditions or satisfy the needs of every patient. For that reason, an elite facial surgery practice or medical spa will recommend the best products available from a variety of manufacturers, but only following a professional skin-care analysis. These recommendations will be based upon what elite skin-care professionals and physicians feel is the most ideal combination of the products deemed necessary to address the specific issues that have been identified.

In compliance with the scientific guidelines used when treating medical conditions, the combination of compounds, their strength within the products, their documented efficacy, and the frequency of use may need to be adjusted in order to obtain the best results *in your case*. Compounding pharmacies can create formulations that address the specific conditions your own skin specialist discovers at the time of your examination.

Ultimately, the best way to keep your skin looking its best is to develop an ongoing professional relationship with an experienced expert trained to care for it and to follow this medically trained professional's recommendations.

Your skin says a lot about you—inside and out. If you do the things required for your skin to look as good as possible, better health is likely to follow.

Whenever some product or technology is developed that will improve my patients' appearance, I call it to their attention. Such has been the case with retinoids, derivatives of vitamin A, and alpha hydroxy acids that produce similar results. In many cases, both can improve very early (and very superficial) facial wrinkling.

As you now know, your skin is constantly renewing itself. New cells are formed in its deeper layer (the dermis). Gradually, these cells move toward the surface. Approximately six weeks later, they become scaly and are shed, rather quickly by young people. As we age, however, the scales accumulate and cause your skin to develop a dull, lifeless appearance. That's where exfoliation products and procedures can help. A level 1 microdermabrasion performed by a trained skin-care specialist is one way to rid your skin of this scaly, lifeless layer. You can also perform a microabrasion at home by using a handheld abrasive sponge each morning or night. Buf-Puf is the brand of sponge that I have found to be the easiest for my patients to use at home. In fact, I use it every morning—and have done so for the past twenty-five years. So has my wife. You should ask your skin-care specialists what degree of coarseness and type of soap or facial cleanser is right for your skin. Following exfoliation, products like Retin-A are able to penetrate a bit more deeply into your skin, therefore making them more effective. However, you should let your skin-care consultant direct you as to the strength and combination of products to use.

A number of other changes also occur as a result of aging. The protective oil glands become sluggish; blood circulation immediately beneath the skin lessens, thereby impairing nutrition, and, as part of the aging process, the skin loses its elasticity because of the ongoing deterioration of its collagen and elastin network. When used properly and for a long enough period of time, Retin-A and alpha hydroxy acids tend to prevent some of these undesirable changes.

Retinoids (products containing retinoic acid) are potent substances and will cause severe reactions on sensitive skin unless diluted to match the specific conditions that the user's skin exhibits. That's why a prescription from a physician is necessary. Most skin-care centers and medical spas provide Retin-A or Tretinoin in diluted forms and gradually increase their strength over a period of time to avoid unfavorable reactions.

Because Retin-A is a prescription item, its continued use must be supervised by a physician. Like any medication, if products that contain retinoic acid are not used as prescribed, they cannot be expected to achieve the results desired.

Alpha hydroxy acids are another class of topical exfoliates. These products are usually available through most medical spas and skin-care centers. Understand that neither Retin-A nor alpha hydroxy acid is a substitute for cosmetic surgery or advanced skin resurfacing performed by a physician. However, they are helpful adjuncts in professionally managed skin care following cosmetic surgery and advanced skin resurfacing.

As a result of improper usage, many patients become disenchanted with skin polishers. One of the most common conditions is intense redness and peeling. This condition most often occurs when full-strength (1 percent) Retin-A is used from a tube. Because of these common—but avoidable—sequelae, most skin experts prefer to start their patients and clients on a product other than Retin-A or on more dilute concentrations. In conjunction with an elite facial surgeon, a professional aesthetician can recommend the most appropriate product and routine for each skin type.

After your skin develops some resistance, the strength of the preparation can be increased with each subsequent prescription. I recommend that you stay with each diluted prescription for three months before increasing the concentration. It is advisable to return for follow-up visits, especially during the first year.

Although some of my patients see improvement in the texture and vitality of their skin early in the course of treatment, the best results are usually not apparent until skin polishers have has been used daily for six to nine months. Unlike a chemical peel, which is a more permanent measure to improve the conditions found in aging skin, it is necessary to continue treatment with skin polishers indefinitely.

Sensible Sun Protection: Facts about Sunscreens

I am often asked, "What can I do to prevent wrinkles and slow down the aging process?" The simple answer is, "Avoid tanning beds, and shield your skin from the damaging rays of the sun by reducing exposure."

My recommendations are based upon strong and conclusive evidence that the most severe premature signs of aging exhibited by the appearance of the skin are brought on by cumulative exposure to the sun, wind, or artificial tanning lights. So, if you wish to delay or prevent the premature appearance of wrinkles, blemishes, and skin cancers, minimize your exposure—and begin to do so early in life.

How Does a Sunscreen Work?

Topically applied sunscreens work by absorbing, reflecting, or scattering ultraviolet light, thereby reducing the amount that reaches your skin. The absorbers are chemical agents, and the reflectors are physical agents. Sunscreens should be applied at least thirty minutes prior to being in the sun. Doing so will reduce the amount of ultraviolet (UV) rays that come into contact with your body. Sunscreens are just that—they screen. But they *do not* totally block all UV rays.

Sunscreens should be reapplied every hour or so, especially if you have been perspiring.

Sunscreens' protective abilities vary according to the ingredients. The following information on that subject is provided for readers with backgrounds in science and chemistry. The important thing for you to know is this: *use these products as directed.*

Some sunscreens, such as those containing octyl methoxycinnamate, octyl salicylate, or homosalate, absorb the most dangerous portions of ultraviolet B (UVB) light. Others, like oxybenzone and titanium dioxide, absorb dangerous UVB as well as the more energetic part of ultraviolet A (UVA), while zinc oxide and avobenzone absorb into the highest portions of the UVA spectrum.

What Is Ultraviolet Radiation?

Ultraviolet radiation (UVR) is simply one form of energy coming from the sun. UV rays are the sun's invisible burning rays—the ones that cause sunburn and, in some cases, skin cancer. There are three types of ultraviolet rays.

UVA: These rays maintain maximum constant intensity throughout the year and penetrate more deeply into the skin's layers than UVB rays. They contribute to premature aging, wrinkling, and sagging and the leathery appearance of overly exposed skin.

UVB: These rays, which are stronger than UVA, are more intense in summer months, at higher altitudes, and closer to the equator. UVB is associated with sunburn, premature aging of the skin, and the development of skin cancer.

UVC: Although the strongest and most dangerous, these rays are normally filtered by the ozone layer and do not reach the earth.

The amount of UV you are exposed to varies with the time of day, the seasons, the altitude, the weather conditions, where you live, your medications, reflective surfaces, and the length of time spent in the sun.

What Is the UV Index?

The Environmental Protection Agency, the National Weather Service, and the Center for Disease Control and Prevention launched the national UV Index, which is issued daily to advise you on the strength of the sun's UV rays in your region. The UV Index was recently updated. It goes from 1 to 11+, with the number indicating the amount of UV radiation reaching the earth's surface during the noon hour at a given location on the earth's surface. The higher the UV Index level, the greater the strength of the sun's UV rays and the faster your skin is likely to burn. The National Weather Service forecasts the UV Index daily in fifty-eight US cities. Check the internet or the local newspaper, TV, or radio to learn the UV Index of your area.

What Is the Sun Protection Factor?

The Sun protection factor (SPF) tells you how long a product is expected to protect your skin from burning. The SPF on the label indicates only the degree of UVB protection. For example, an SPF 5 sunscreen should protect your skin from developing redness five times longer than no sunscreen at all, while an SPF 15 product should protect your skin 15 times longer than if no sunscreen were applied. However, the degree of protection offered by a sunscreen depends not only on its concentration but also on how thickly—and how often—you apply it. Therefore, you should apply sunscreen generously, uniformly, and frequently when the occasion calls for it, and you should rub it in. This is particularly important if you are getting in and out of the water or perspiring heavily. Remember to apply the first layer of sunscreen at least thirty minutes prior to exposure. It takes time for the protection to take full effect.

How Should You Choose a Sunscreen?

Your choice of sunscreen should be based on four factors:
- Your skin type.
- The length of time you spend in the sun.

- The intensity of the sun's rays in your geographic area.
- The type of formulation you prefer.

Based on your sunburn and tanning history, the US Food and Drug Administration recommends SPF ranges representing five categories of protection:

- Always burns easily, rarely tans: SPF 20 to 30
- Always burns easily, tans minimally: SPF 12 to under 20
- Burns moderately, tans gradually: SPF 8 to under 12
- Burns minimally, always tans well: SPF 4 to under 8
- Rarely burns, tans profusely: SPF 2 to under 4

Another important point to remember is that the darker your skin, the less likely you are to burn. Melanin, the pigment in the deeper layers of the skin, is a natural reflector of the sun's damaging rays. That's why it is rare to see people of African ancestry with wrinkles and skin cancers. People who are descended from Mediterranean or Central or South American ancestors also have more protective pigment in their skin than people whose ancestors hailed from Northern Europe.

The preceding information is provided to stress that a great deal of research has gone into the science of sun protection. For the average consumer, the following are the key points to remember.

- When purchasing a sunscreen, check the label to make sure your sunscreen protects against UVA and UVB rays (i.e., provides broad-spectrum protection).
- Be alert for sunscreen allergies, especially in the eye or cheekbone area, which might show up as redness, itching, or stinging. If this occurs, wash off the sunscreen product with a mild soap, and apply topical cortisone. If your eyes or tongue begin to swell, take twenty-five milligrams of Benadryl. If the swelling does not begin to subside within thirty minutes, consult a physician.
- As a rule, sunscreens with microfine titanium dioxide or zinc oxide are less likely to cause an allergic reaction.

- Certain medications—including diuretics, many antibiotics (such as sulfas and tetracyclines), antidepressants, and some birth control pills—can make your skin more sensitive to sunlight. Therefore, exposure to UV rays might lead to an increase in the frequency of adverse reactions to these drugs.
- High-risk individuals, such as those who have sun-damaged skin, an autoimmune disease, brown spots, or a history of skin cancer, should wear a sunscreen that has the best UVA and UVB protection if they are going to be exposed to intense sun.

When and How Should I Use a Sunscreen?

Because of their importance, I wish to emphasize some of the instructions mentioned earlier in this chapter. Sunscreens should be applied (by rubbing them into your skin) about thirty minutes before every exposure to the sun and reapplied frequently and liberally, using about an ounce to cover your entire body, at least every two hours for as long as you are exposed to the sun.

Because sunscreen products differ in their degrees of water resistance, they should always be reapplied after swimming, sweating, or rubbing the skin with towels or tissue paper.

Don't forget to apply sunscreen to all exposed skin, including your lips, nose, ears, neck, scalp, hands, feet, and other areas that are especially prone to sunburn. Once your skin starts to burn, get out of the sun. Don't reapply the sunscreen in hopes that it will keep your skin from burning. It won't! And remember, 70–80 percent of the sun's damaging rays can penetrate through clouds and water, so you need to use a sunscreen under these conditions as well.

Expert Advice

The daily use of an effective sunscreen definitely qualifies as a gift you can give yourself. Disciplined use of sun protection as described in this chapter can help reduce your chances of premature aging, premature wrinkling, and skin cancer. Most experts agree, however, that if you can avoid the sun between the hours of 10:00 a.m. and 4:00 p.m., do so. If you must be exposed—regardless of the time of day—use the protective measures recommended here.

CHAPTER 27

Treating Skin Cancer

Types of Skin Cancer

Repeated and prolonged exposure to ultraviolet light, whether from sun exposure or from tanning beds, can be damaging to the skin. The effects of these damaging rays are cumulative over a lifetime. The more exposure a person gets, the higher their chances of eventually getting some form of skin cancer. The fairer their complexion, the greater their risk, whereas individuals with dark or black skin have a much lower risk. Suntan lotions with an SPF greater than fifteen can help protect the skin and should always be used prior to any sun exposure—and reapplied frequently.

There are three major types of skin cancer: basal cell, squamous cell, and melanoma.

The most common form is basal cell carcinoma, which is primarily found on the face or other exposed areas of the body. It is usually raised and pink with pearly borders and might crust or bleed as it enlarges. It has a tendency to grow very slowly and invade local structures, such as the nose, lips, or eyes. It almost never spreads (metastasizes) to any distant areas of the body but can cause significant local damage if not treated early. Early surgical cure is almost 99 percent effective. Sclerosing or morpheaform basal cell carcinomas are not usually raised above the skin, as seen with rodent ulcer basal cell cancers. The former tend to grow like the roots of an oak tree, surfacing and diving underneath the surface.

Squamous cell carcinoma is usually found on exposed areas of the body, such as the scalp, ears, and lips, but can occur elsewhere. It is usually raised and pink with irregular edges, and it commonly ulcerates or becomes crusty in the center. It has a greater tendency to metastasize than basal cell carcinoma, but again, if treated early, it has an excellent chance for complete cure.

Melanoma can arise on any area of the body. It is usually a brown, black, or multicolored patch or plaque with an irregular border, and it might have satellite spots of a similar nature surrounding the larger lesion. In rare cases, melanomas are not pigmented. Melanomas can originate in a preexisting mole or occur as an isolated lesion. Any change in the appearance of a mole is highly suspicious. Melanoma has a high rate of metastasis if not treated early and is perhaps the most dangerous form of skin cancer.

If you have any moles or skin growths that you are concerned about, it is best to have your doctor examine these. Any growth that is suspicious should be biopsied to rule out the possibility of a cancer. Remember, if treated early, almost all skin cancers are curable.

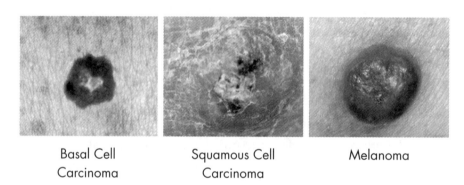

| Basal Cell Carcinoma | Squamous Cell Carcinoma | Melanoma |

Mohs Micrographic Surgery

Mohs surgery is a form of surgical excision that provides for an accurate assessment of the completeness of tumor removal. As a result, it has a very high cure rate and can spare more tissue than conventional surgery, thus resulting in less scarring. The Mohs technique requires that the surgeon be able to microscopically evaluate the excised tissue. As a result, this type of surgery requires special equipment and training and can be more expensive and time-consuming than conventional surgery. Thus, Mohs surgery is usually reserved for those instances in which it is very important to preserve normal skin—such as surgeries around the eyes, nose, lips, or ears—or in which other types of treatments have either failed or would not be as successful.

Electrodessication and Curettage (ED&C)

An older method of treating skin cancer consists of scraping (curettage) and burning with an electrical current (electrodesiccating) of the visible and palpable tumor and some surrounding skin. This procedure does not provide a method of assessing whether the tumor has been completely destroyed. It usually results in a circular wound that heals with a circular scar in three to eight weeks. It should be used only to treat primary skin cancer—that is, skin cancer that has never been previously treated—and should not be used on certain body sites.

Surgical Excision

This method provides for the removal of a skin cancer and the subsequent repair of the wound created. It also provides tissue for microscopic assessment of the completeness of tumor removal. However, the usual laboratory techniques used to assess this process of tumor removal, although good, are not complete; however, they are adequate for the majority of tumors. Surgical excision usually heals in one to two weeks with a linear or geometric scar, depending on the extent of surgery required. However, depending on the nature of the tumor, some patients could require extensive reconstruction. After the scars are mature (usually within twelve to eighteen months), additional plastic surgery can be used to improve or camouflage them. (See chapter 28.) Surgery for skin cancers is usually an outpatient procedure performed under local anesthesia.

Cryosurgery

Cryosurgery destroys skin cancer by utilizing intense cold in the form of liquid nitrogen. Like ED&C, this method does not provide for assessment of complete tumor removal. Ideally, it should be performed with the use of cryoprobes (needles inserted into the skin to measure temperature changes) in order to obtain optimal destruction of the tumor. It usually heals in a manner similar to electrodessication and curettage.

Radiation Therapy

Another method of destroying skin cancer utilizes specifically controlled radiation energy. It is useful in those patients who would not be able to tolerate surgical procedures, either because of medical problems or because of fear of surgery. It is also useful in those anatomical locations that would necessitate extensive reconstruction. It can be used to treat primary tumors; however, it does not provide for assessment of the completeness of tumor removal. Healing takes place over four to eight weeks, usually with a good cosmetic response. However, some patients can develop significant scarring and radiation damage of the skin. Occasionally, the radiation can cause the development of a new skin cancer in the area of the previous treatment many years later. Because the tissues have been previously exposed to radiation, healing from surgical therapy often becomes less predictable. Radiation therapy is usually performed over a period of three to five weeks.

Mohs Micrographic Surgery:
The State-of-the-Art Method of Treating Skin Cancer

I previously referred to a technique known as Mohs micrographic surgery. Among the various modalities of removing skin cancer, this is considered by most experts to be the gold standard.

Dr. Frederic Mohs of the University of Wisconsin developed this technique nearly fifty years ago. It offers patients the highest chance of cure with maximal preservation of normal tissue, thereby reducing the difficulty of reconstructing defects that result from tumor removal. However, because his method was viewed as a threat by those who performed the other procedures previously described in this chapter, Dr. Mohs was ostracized by those segments of his profession. It is not an uncommon story. Years later, however, Dr. Fred Mohs is credited with revolutionizing the treatment of skin cancer—and rightly so.

It is true that his method is time consuming, requires highly specialized training, and is not always necessary for treating skin cancer. In fact, only a small number of dermatologists in the United States are equipped to offer such treatment.

There are three surgical steps to treating skin cancer with Mohs micrographic surgery.

1. Surgical removal of the visible portion of the skin cancer.
2. Surgical removal of a thin layer of tissue at the bed and periphery of the cancer, with meticulous mapping and color coding of the tissue.
3. Immediate examination of this excised tissue under a microscope, using the mapping to determine the extent of the tumor and whether there is a need for further surgery.

If residual cancer is detected, a Mohs surgeon is able to locate the remaining cancer, and steps two through three are repeated until the tumor is completely removed.

This surgery is usually performed under local anesthesia as an outpatient. The actual surgery usually takes fifteen to thirty minutes per stage of tissue removal, after which a temporary bandage is placed on the wound. The excised tissue is then prepared for microscopic evaluation in a process that can take up to an hour. During this time, you may wait in the waiting room. If the evaluation reveals that your tissue still contains cancer cells, the procedure will be repeated as soon as possible. Several excisions and microscopic examinations might need to be done in one day; rarely, the process might require two days. However, the average number of surgical stages for most skin cancers is two or three, meaning that most patients have their entire skin cancer removed by midday on the day of surgery. You should plan on spending the entire day at the surgeon's office, so bring something to do or read.

Will the Surgery Leave a Scar?

Yes; any form of therapy will leave a scar. We make every effort to obtain the optimal cosmetic result for you, but the primary emphasis is on removal or destruction of your skin cancer, and because of the variability of individual healing, the final scar cannot be accurately predicted or controlled. In many cases, additional plastic surgery can improve the scars that remain. In more complicated cases, a plastic surgeon may be requested to repair the defect at the time of cancer removal.

What Are the Risks of Mohs Surgery?

The risks are the same as those associated with other surgeries of a similar nature. They include allergic reactions to anesthesia, bleeding, infection, scarring, and an unsatisfactory response. In addition, there might be certain risks associated with your own unique situation, influenced by the location of the tumor and any other medical problems you have. There is also always a possibility that additional treatments might be necessary.

The Surgical Wound

When the skin cancer has been completely removed, a decision is then made regarding the appropriate method for treating or reconstructing the wound that has been created. The usual choices include:

1. Letting the wound heal by itself (granulation).
2. Closing the wound with stitches (primary repair).
3. Closing the wound with a flap (moving skin around) or a graft (transplanting skin from one body site to another).
4. Delayed closure of the wound with the above choices.

The method used will be determined by the nature, extent, and location of the tumor and the resultant wound. We will recommend which method is best suited in your case. The most appropriate method of repair is usually apparent before performing Mohs surgery, but on occasion, the exact nature and extent of the tumor and resultant wound will not be apparent until afterward. However, the recommended treatment plan is always discussed with the patient before proceeding with it. Surgical repair is usually performed in the afternoon after the Mohs surgery is completed.

If the wound is allowed to heal by itself (granulation), it usually heals over four to eight weeks. If one of the other methods, besides delayed closure, is used, it usually heals in one to two weeks.

Your doctor or surgeon will provide the appropriate posttreatment instructions for you. You are strongly urged to follow them. By faithfully adhering to your doctor's orders, you give yourself the best chance of healing quickly and minimizing scarring.

All wounds can initially be faintly red and slightly tender, itch, drain clear fluid, and show some swelling that disappears gradually. However, persistence or an increase in these signs and symptoms can indicate a problem, such as infection, and should be brought to your doctor's attention.

Most patients do not complain of pain following skin cancer surgery. After your surgical area heals, you might notice a red scar that gradually fades. The scar can be elevated or depressed initially but usually flattens. Sometimes the scar can be sensitive to touch or temperature or can have altered sensations such as itching or numbness, which usually improve with time. However, unless treated with injections of cortisone, some of these changes outlined above can be permanent.

What If I Don't Like the Scar?

If you find the final scar to be unsatisfactory, there are various treatments that can be attempted in order to modify the scar. In any event, we recommend that you wait twelve to eighteen months before seeking modification of a scar, since scars undergo their own biological modification. However, in some cases, cortisone injections or dermabrasion can provide improvement within six weeks following surgery. I have not found the topical application of commercially available antiscarring products to be any more effective than the tincture of time and the treatment modalities addressed above.

Follow-Up Surgery?

A follow-up period of at least five years is necessary after a cancer-removal wound has healed. Experience has shown that recurrence usually occurs within the first year of surgery and that once you develop a skin cancer, there is a possibility you will develop others. The reason is that the surrounding areas have been subjected to the same factors (sun and wind damage) that created the cancer you had treated.

For this reason, you will be asked to return for a follow-up exam of your skin and the surgical site after six months, after one year, and annually for at least five years. If you were referred by another physician, this follow-up can be performed by them. Any suspicious area should be evaluated at once.

What about Exposure to the Sun?

Chapter 26 of this book addresses sun protection. Please refer to it and heed its recommendations.

Terms that relate to Skin Cancer Diagnoses and Treatment

- **Benign/Malignant:** A benign tumor invades nearby tissue but will not spread throughout the body, whereas a malignant tumor might.
- **Biopsy:** The removal of tissue from the living body for the purpose of evaluating the tissue microscopically in order to determine the nature and extent of a pathological, unhealthy, or diseased process. Usually, a biopsy consists only of a part of the disease process (i.e., a small part of a tumor).
- **Cancer:** A general term for many different diseases characterized by an abnormal and uncontrolled growth of cells that can invade and destroy surrounding normal tissues. Certain types of cancer also have the ability to spread (metastasize) through the blood or lymph nodes to start new cancers in other body parts.
- **Keratoses:** Nonmalignant skin lesions that can be nonpigmented or deeply pigmented, are scaly to the touch, and are present for longer than six weeks.
- **Lesion:** Any new growth or mass that appears on your skin or within your body.

- **Lymph Nodes:** Small, round "peanut-like" structures in the body that act as filters to stop the spread of disease. Inflammations of these filtering bodies are often referred to as kernels.
- **Nevus (Mole):** A benign tumor of the skin that can be present at birth or appear after birth. There is a possibility that some moles can go on to become a type of skin cancer.
- **Pathology (Micrographic Assessment):** The evaluation of tissue under the microscope in order to assess the type of disease process (cancer) or the extent of disease involvement.
- **Tumor:** A localized growth of cells. A tumor can be benign (a non-cancerous growth that does not destroy and spread) or malignant (a growth of cancer cells).

What Are the Causes of Skin Cancer?

As with other types of cancer, the cause of skin cancer is not completely known. As explained in other sections of this book, excessive exposure to sunlight is the single most important factor associated with development of skin cancers. Fair-skinned individuals develop skin cancer more frequently than dark-skinned individuals. Skin cancer also tends to be hereditary and occurs very frequently in certain ethnic groups, especially those with fair complexions, such as people from Northern Europe. Other possible causes of skin cancer include X-rays, trauma, and certain chemicals.

Reconstruction of Cancer Defects

After the removal of skin cancers or some instances of traumatic injury, there is insufficient tissue to close the wound or fill the defect. In these cases, it might be necessary to borrow some skin, bone, or cartilage from another area of the body in order to reconstruct the missing tissues. This is commonly done by using either a graft or a flap.

A graft is a portion of tissue that is completely removed from the body and transferred to a different area. It has been separated from its blood supply, and therefore, once transferred, it is necessary for new capillaries to grow into the graft to feed it the nutrients required for its survival. Grafts are limited in their size, since the new blood vessels can only carry these nutrients a very short distance.

On the other hand, a flap is a portion of tissue that remains attached to the body at some location, is "hinged" at this attachment, and is moved into the defect area. Since the flap is never separated from its blood supply, larger amounts of tissue can be transferred more reliably. In some instances, it is possible to disconnect a large flap from its blood supply, move it to another place on the body, and microscopically reattach it to another set of blood vessels.

This is known as a free flap and is understandably more complex and less reliable than a simple flap. Sometimes, however, these flaps present the best method of reconstruction.

If you do not have sufficient tissue to transfer, it can occasionally be necessary to use a graft of tissue (usually cartilage or bone) from another person to correct a defect. This tissue can be obtained from a tissue bank. Due to the body's immune system, it is not possible to take living skin from one person and transplant it to another person; however, cartilage and bone, if properly prepared, can be transferred.

Sometimes, it may be possible to stretch the available skin by placing a medical-grade balloon or expander under the skin and gradually inflating it to stretch the overlying skin. This is usually done in two operations performed about six to eight weeks apart. During the interval between operations, the expander is incrementally inflated every two to three days until there is sufficient skin to reconstruct the defect.

During the second operation, the inflated expander is removed, and reconstruction is carried out. In order to correct a complicated defect, it may be necessary to use many of these techniques. Your surgeon will discuss the particular techniques that they feel best suit your problem prior to surgery.

Tissue expanders are frequently used in surgery designed to reconstruct the breasts following cancer surgery.

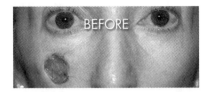
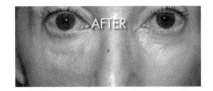
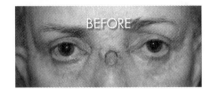
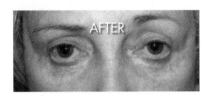

The defect seen in the preoperative photographs resulted from removal of skin cancers by the Mohs technique. Reconstruction of the defects were performed in single operations by shifting surrounding tissues into the defects.

CHAPTER 28

Scar Revision and Skin Surgery

The previous chapter dealt with measures a body owner can take to prevent and treat skin cancers. While some topical skin cancer remedies are promising, surgical excision along with microscopic examination of the excised margins remains the gold standard. In some cases, concisely focused radiation can destroy cancerous cells in the skin as well as underneath. However, scars can also occur from noncancerous conditions, such as surgical incisions, injuries, and infections.

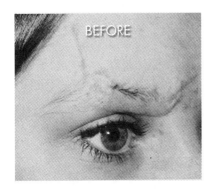 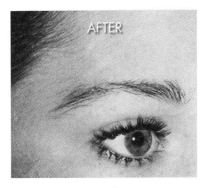

The scars in this young woman were the result of an automobile accident. Three stages of correction were required in order to help them blend into her uninjured skin.

Unsightly, disfiguring scars can be disconcerting and often devastating to one's self-image. In addition to scars, other blemishes or defects that can be removed or improved with carefully planned plastic surgical techniques include keratoses (age spots), moles, birthmarks, and cysts.

Keratoses and some moles might require only a superficial shave followed by light cauterization of the base. In most cases, no visible scar is created.

Other lesions may be completely excised with surgery. However, when all layers of the skin are penetrated, a scar will result. While tiny

202 | The Gift You Give Yourself

defects can be allowed to heal on their own (secondary intention), most must be repaired by advancing the raw edges together (primary closure) or through skin grafts or flaps of adjacent skin. It is important for you to remember that any time an incision or injury penetrates all layers of the skin, some scarring will result. In most situations, additional revisionary surgery within six to twelve months can help provide a more satisfactory result. However, in children a longer period of scar maturation is required. This is one of the factual paradoxes that surgeons and parents alike are forced to accept and deal with.

The appearance of most scars or blemishes can be improved by well-planned and carefully executed surgery, but there are some important facts patients contemplating such procedures should know. Scars are usually unsightly when they:

- Are wide.
- Are longer than one inch.
- Cross natural creases or facial contour lines.
- Are elevated above the adjacent skin.
- Are depressed below the adjacent skin.
- Are a different color than adjacent tissues.

If any or all of the above characteristics are present, improvement in any one of them should make the scars less conspicuous. As demonstrated in the following photographs, correction of two or three of these factors can often result in dramatic improvement of the appearance (and sometimes the function) of the scarring.

Injections of cortisone preparations directly into a thick, elevated, painful scar or a scar that itches can often provide dramatic improvement. For best results, these injections should be repeated every three weeks until the activity within the scar is arrested. To help my patients understand how cortisone improves the appearance of thick, painful scars, I use the following example. Cortisone injected directly into such a scar cools hot spots from which new—and unnecessary—tissue is being created, just as pouring water on a fire douses the flames. Not until enough water has been poured on the fire to cool the coals is the possibility of a new fire nonexistent. In like manner, cortisone must be injected into a hypertrophic scar or keloid every three weeks until its hot spots are cooled.

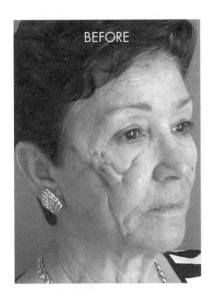
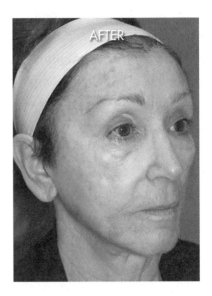

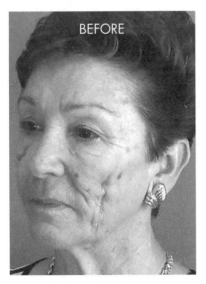
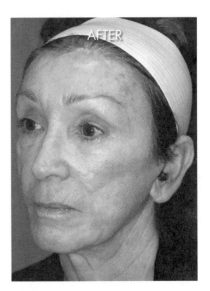

The scars on this woman were the result of an infection that occurred following fat injections to her face performed by another surgeon. Her scars were excised and revised with a series of surgical maneuvers.

Surgical treatment for deep scars and skin defects implies that incisions will be made to remove the existing scar or blemish and replace it with one that is less conspicuous.

Here's a truth that must not be overlooked or forgotten. Each incision made into the skin—regardless of where it is placed, who makes it, for what purpose it is made, or whether it is deliberate or accidental—heals in the same manner as any other cut. That is, it produces scar tissue—nature's method of healing. This simple fact is frequently forgotten or ignored by individuals who think that a plastic surgeon can make an incision leaving no visible scar or can, in fact, eliminate existing scars.

In reality, the surgeon's goal is to replace an unsightly or disfiguring scar with a better scar—one that is more narrow and more level, blends with the surrounding skin surface, and causes no contracture or pull on the surrounding structures. In short, one that is as inconspicuous as possible. The final appearance, however, is dependent on many factors, one of which is the patient's own healing capability.

You might be someone who, possibly due to conditioning by what you've seen on television and in the movies, expects the final result of a healing wound to occur rapidly. Unless duly informed, you will also be disappointed and troubled because you must wait for nature to take its course—that is, for the maturation process to run its course. Maturation is the continuing change in appearance all scars progress through until they reach a state where no further change will occur.

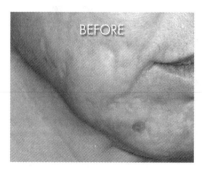 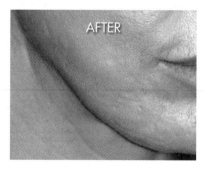

The scars on this young woman's face were caused by cystic acne. A series of carefully placed surgical incision removed the existing scars. Dermabrasion was performed a few months later.

Full maturation of scars can take from six to eighteen months or sometimes longer, especially in young children. Initially, a freshly repaired incision of scar usually looks pretty good. As the healing process moves forward, the scar will become reddened, possibly somewhat raised above the surrounding skin, and frequently hard or lumpy. Gradually, unless your scar is frequently stressed by stretching the surrounding skin, its firmness and red color should lessen and disappear, leaving a softer scar that is usually more level with and somewhat lighter in color than the adjacent skin. In some cases, injection of cortisone preparations directly into or underneath the scar can speed up the process.

NATURE'S HAND IN HEALING

Following an injury most patients wish to have surgical correction of scars immediately. This case demonstrates that waiting can sometimes be the best treatment.

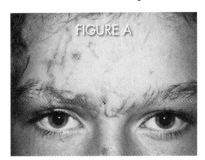

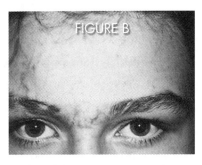

Figure A shows scarring of the forehead shortly after an accident.

Figure B shows some improvement three months later without any treatment.

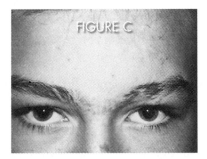

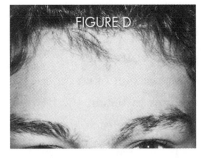

Figure C shows that the lumps have flattened and the deep pink or red color has diminished six months later.

Figure D shows the area has healed nicely with minimal scarring approximately two years later. No surgery was performed.

Patients seeking scar revision should be emotionally prepared to accept several facts. First, removal will result in another scar, though hopefully an improved one. Second, the final appearance will not be evident for six to eighteen months. Third, more than one procedure might be required. This brings us to another very important matter. Understandably, most people with recent scarring want repairs immediately; however, except in select cases, scar revision should not be undertaken too soon following the initial repair of the wound. The passage of time is the best, the kindest, and, in the long run, the simplest treatment to give to any scar of recent origin, as most will undergo spontaneous improvement if given enough time to do so—often six to eighteen months.

Only after a scar has become soft and white is it mature. A decision regarding a second-stage revision may be delayed until this time has elapsed. However, since little or no improvement in the basic problem can be anticipated with the passage of time, scars that cause distortion of normal structures (eyebrows, lips, eyelids, nostrils, etc.), scars that spread widely or produce deformity by contraction, and U- or J-shaped scars may be repaired earlier. When removing an existing scar or blemish by excision, the surgeon makes every effort to place the line of incision as nearly as possible in or parallel to one of the normal crease lines of the face or body. Sometimes it may be necessary to change the direction of a scar so that it will follow these lines.

Excision of large, unsightly scars, birthmarks, or blemishes can require multiple operations over a period of time (serial excisions). Occasionally, it is necessary to shift surrounding tissue to fill a defect or, rarely, to even resort to skin grafting.

Scar revision often requires at least two (frequently three) surgical procedures to obtain the best achievable result. Usually, six to twelve months separate each stage. Some scars mature more quickly, meaning subsequent stages can be performed sooner. It bears repeating that in children and adolescents, maturation of scars can take eighteen to twenty-four months, sometimes longer, while the same scar on a patient in their sixties or older might be flat, thin, and soft within three months.

This is one of the unpredictable factors that accounts for the variability in the final result that occurs with scar revision and wound healing.

The following section deals with appearance-enhancing procedures beyond the face, nose, head, and neck. Although the vast majority of body-contouring procedures are performed on women, men comprise a rapidly growing segment of candidates.

CHAPTER 29

Surgical Body Contouring

In the previous chapters, we have primarily focused on procedures and products designed to enhance the features above your shoulders. Now we move on to other regions of your body and explore ways to enhance them.

As stated at the outset, I am a facial plastic surgeon and personally perform surgeries only of the head and neck. However, during my training, I was exposed to and assisted with plastic surgical procedures on other parts of the body. In addition, I have had plastic surgeons working in my clinics for the past thirty years. Many times, I perform a facial or nasal procedure at the same time one of my associates or partners is performing a procedure on the body. Therefore, I am more than familiar with breast- and body-sculpting procedures. The body-focused cases presented in the following chapters were performed by my plastic surgery associates, some of whom contributed to the information I share with you.

Few people are born with a perfectly proportioned body. Even those who possessed the near-perfect bodies of youth see them change for the worse as years pass. The good news is that, through the miracles of modern medicine and surgery, it is possible to improve upon the body that nature gave you and on which time has taken a toll. "Made-to-order" procedures are designed to enhance the size and shape of a variety of anatomical areas.

Medical-grade implants are often used to provide women who have smaller-than-desired breasts the look and shape they dream of. Intelligent liposuction can help reduce the size of larger-than-optimal thighs, hips, and "saddlebags" in men and women. But there is more. By firming and building muscle through reasonable exercise programs, maintaining the hormones of youth at an optimal level (or returning them to that level), and ingesting the appropriate proportions and types of foods and supplements, you will be able to even further enhance the improvements made by breast- and body-sculpting surgery.

When, after the age of fifty, someone loses more than fifty pounds, it is generally necessary to remove sagging skin with surgery, especially in the neck and abdominal regions. Women in this age group and those who lose large amounts of weight generally benefit from breast lifting as well. Both men and women might also require removal of excess skin in the hips and thighs. There is one exception: since youthful skin tends to shrink following weight loss and liposuction, many younger patients (under the age of forty) might not require skin excision at the time of liposuction.

Breast Augmentation

Breast augmentation or augmentation mammaplasty is the plastic surgical procedure used to increase the size and shape of a woman's breast. This is accomplished by the placement of medical-grade implants underneath the natural breast tissue.

Breast augmentation is the second most common surgical enhancement performed. Only liposuction tops it. Enhancing the size and appearance of a woman's breast can be psychologically rewarding and can go a long way toward improving her self-image, as it did in the case of the young woman whose photographs are shared below.

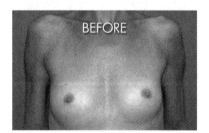 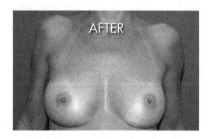

Photos courtesy of Dr. Brentley Taylor.

An important part of the preoperative consultation should include a general determination of the desired breast size. Although almost any degree of augmentation can be achieved, you and your surgeon must decide on a general improvement that coincides with your total body size and shape in addition to your preoperative breast size. Your ultimate breast size will be determined at the time of operation.

To accomplish the most attractive and natural-appearing results, the implants must be carefully placed within a pocket the surgeon creates beneath the existing breast tissue.

Implants can be placed under the muscle (in the submuscular plane) or on top of the muscle and directly underneath the breast gland. Your surgeon will perform an extensive evaluation of your breasts, noting the skin quality, the breast tissue thickness, and the degree of sagging. Recommendations as to which approach is best for you are totally customized and are based on the above criteria as well as on other factors that will be addressed by the surgeon you choose. Some advantages to subglandular placement (on top of the muscles of your chest) include a quicker recovery and a more natural appearance. Some advantages of submuscular placement (under the muscle) are a slightly decreased risk of capsular contraction (firmness of the breast) and slightly better imaging when mammography is performed for cancer screening.

As with any surgical procedure, incisions must be made into the skin in order to place your implants. Your incisions can be placed beneath the breast (inframammary), hidden in the skin crease. Implants can also be inserted via an incision within the armpit (axilla) or around the areola part of the nipple complex. The inframammary approach is the most common approach used. The scars in the thinner skin of the anterior armpit, however, are virtually imperceptible. Regardless of the incision, every effort is made to obtain the best scar possible. Your overall health, your healing capacity, and how well you follow your postoperative instructions help determine how well your scars will or will not heal.

As with other appearance-enhancing procedures, the most attractive breasts are ones on which signs of surgery are not present. A common—and avoidable—mistake is for either the patient or the surgeon to recommend implants that are too large for the patient's body composition. In addition, the dreaded capsular formation (or hardening) of the breasts seems to occur more in cases where large implants were placed. Although I do not personally perform breast augmentation, my facial and nasal patients often ask my advice. This is what I tell them:

212 | The Gift You Give Yourself

"Whatever implant size your surgeon recommends, insist on one size smaller." Those who followed my advice often thank me. Those who do not often tell me they wish they had. As with noses, chins, faces, and eyelids, extremes are to be avoided!

Several options of anesthesia are available for breast augmentation, including "twilight sleep" with local injection or general anesthesia. In most cases, my associates use the patient's preference. Some patients find that the submuscular implant placement is a bit uncomfortable and that the period of convalescence is several days longer than when a subglandular operation is performed.

Because breast augmentation is a surgical procedure, you need to consider many of the complications associated with any other surgery. Reactions to medications, poor scarring, hematoma, and infection are possible with any surgery, and several potential complications are unique to breast augmentation. Asymmetry or improper location of the implants is possible. The incidence of asymmetry is more common when there is preoperative discrepancy in the size of the breasts. Surgeons attempt to obtain symmetry by using implants of different sizes, but asymmetry might sometimes persist.

One of the most common problems associated with breast augmentation is temporary loss of nipple sensation. Loss of nipple sensation is almost always transitory and eventually resolves. Permanent loss of sensation is unusual but can occur anywhere in the breast. The other most common problem is the formation of scar tissue "capsules" that cause the breast to feel hard to the touch. Capsules are circumferential scars that develop around the implants, causing an unnatural firmness to the breast. Although submuscular placement of the implants has decreased the incidence of this problem, some degree of firmness is occasionally present.

If the capsule should become severe, causing an unnatural-appearing or painful breast, a second operation to release the capsule might be necessary. Postsurgical massage of implanted breasts is an important step in preventing capsule formation.

Mastopexy: The Breast-Lift Procedure

Mastopexy is the operation designed to reposition or lift breasts that have become ptotic (drooping). Breast ptosis most commonly results from volume loss following pregnancy and nursing or after a large weight gain and loss. The volume of breast tissue decreases, leaving behind a skin envelope that is too large for the glandular tissue within, thus allowing the nipple and remaining breast tissue to sag much lower than normal. Once the process of sagging begins, the breast shape and contour never return to their more erect, youthful appearance on their own. Surgery is the only option. To reposition the nipple and breast tissue, skin incisions are required. The excess skin must be removed and the nipple and areola moved upward to a more attractive and natural position over the remaining breast tissue. This improves the chest and breast contour while maintaining breast size. Since breasts sag as a result of some degree of shrinkage (involution) of the breast tissue, breast augmentation with an implant can be a useful adjunct to the mastopexy operation. General anesthesia is usually required for mastopexy.

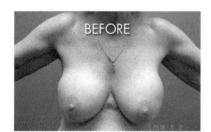 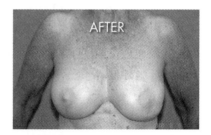

Photos courtesy of Dr. Brentley Taylor.

The convalescence for breast lifting is similar to breast augmentation and requires limited activity for three weeks and a support bra for three months. Due to the extent of the incisions necessary for mastopexy, attention to postoperative care on the part of the patient facilitates the best possible healing of the scars. It is not unusual to have a portion of the scar heal less well and require revision via an office procedure at a later date. Just as with facelift and eyelid operations in which extensive incisions are necessary, the surgeon makes every attempt to hide the incisions and make them as inconspicuous as possible.

Complications specifically related to mastopexy include asymmetric nipple placement and size discrepancies, especially when these conditions existed preoperatively. Infection, scarring, and loss of the nipple or nipple sensation—although rare—can occur. Avoiding any form of nicotine for a minimum of two weeks prior to and after surgery gives the patient the best chance to heal well and minimize scarring.

Breast Reduction Surgery: Reduction Mammaplasty for Women and Men

Reduction mammaplasty, or breast reduction, is the name given to the surgical reduction of abnormally large breasts. In this procedure, excess breast tissue and breast skin are removed, and the nipple is repositioned into a more normal and attractive location.

An infrequently appreciated fact is that men's breast enlarge with aging. This is because of decreased production of the male hormone (testosterone) and the greater impact the female hormone (estrogen, which all men produce in small amounts) has on male breast tissue. Yes, all men have breast tissue, just to a much lesser degree than women. With age, however, even this small amount of breast tissue can cause the glandular material in a man's breast to enlarge. For men, large breasts are a source of embarrassment and unsightliness. For women with large, pendulous breasts, the condition is equally embarrassing but can also lead to other health conditions.

The excess weight of large, sagging breasts can produce chronic neck and shoulder discomfort. Over time, deep creases develop in the skin of a woman's shoulders as a result of her bra straps pressing into the tissues. As a result of these conditions, reduction mammaplasty might be covered by one's health-insurance policy. A preoperative consultation with a surgeon who specializes in breast surgery will include an inventory of the problems related to large, heavy breasts, including neck pain, back pain, raw areas under the breasts (dermatitis), and breast pain.

Dense, heavy breast tissue also makes it more difficult to examine the breast for cancerous changes. Women of all ages who suffer from these problems in addition to the cosmetic and figure-related deformities caused by large breasts are candidates for breast reduction.

Surgery for breast reduction requires more extensive incisions than mastopexy (breast lifting) or breast augmentation. These incisions are required to reduce the volume of the breast tissue as well as to reduce the skin envelope of the reduced breast size.

As with mastopexy, the nipple and areola must be lifted to a more normal position and centered over the remaining breast tissue. These incisions are carefully designed to be hidden in the natural creases and shadows of the breast. Normally, scars mature and become less apparent after several months. To reduce the tension on the incisions and to help alleviate the discomfort that the weight even of smaller breasts causes on suture lines, a support bra is recommended. Antitension skin tapes can be used to support the skin edges around suture lines and to further assist in preventing scars from becoming wide and thick. Patients usually find that a support bra increases postoperative comfort for several months.

Complications specifically related to breast reduction include asymmetries in nipple and breast size, collection of serum and blood beneath the incisions, and, occasionally, prolonged scabbing of the incisions. In very large breasts with a large nipple movement, there is a possibility of nipple or skin loss. The likelihood of this potential problem increases in patients who exhibit total body obesity or who consume nicotine, whether through smoking, snuff usage, e-cigarettes, patches, or gums. In fact, many surgeons will refuse to perform this procedure on patients whose blood tests positive for nicotine.

Prior to consultation, patients undergoing breast reduction must carefully consider what their goals are, and they must have a good idea as to their desired breast size. This will allow the patient and the surgeon to pursue a common objective and for the results obtained through surgery to be more in keeping with what is expected.

An extremely high level of satisfaction is typical for women who undergo breast reduction. In fact, it has been said that these are the happiest and most grateful segment of the patients who choose to give themselves the gift that—more often than not—keeps on giving: appearance- and health-enhancing surgery.

General anesthesia is necessary for breast reduction. Depending upon a patient's total body weight and breast size prior to surgery, a blood transfusion might be indicated. If your surgeon anticipates the need for a blood transfusion, you might be asked to have a unit of your own blood drawn and stowed away at a blood bank at least two weeks prior to surgery. The donated blood may or may not be given back at the time of operation. If you are contemplating breast reduction, know that while the need for blood transfusions is possible, it is rarely required. Even so, overnight hospitalization is usually required with breast reduction procedures. This will be discussed at the time of your consultation. If your health-insurance plan agrees to cover the cost of the surgery, hospitalization costs are usually covered as well.

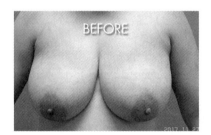 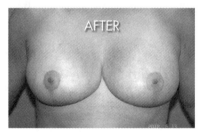

Photos courtesy of Dr. Brentley Taylor.

CHAPTER 30

Beyond the Breasts

The forty-three-year-old woman in the photographs below wished to improve the contour of her abdomen, hips, and thighs in order to give herself more confidence and allow her to wear more fashionable clothes. This is a story commonly seen by appearance-enhancing surgeons. In her case, a combination of techniques was used, including a tummy tuck and thigh lift with liposuction. Her surgical scar was hidden under her panty line and would continue to fade over the next twelve to sixteen months.

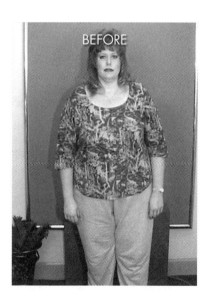 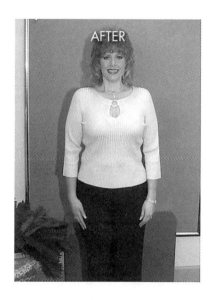

Liposuction—the removal of unwanted fat in certain parts of the body—is now the most commonly performed plastic surgery in the United States. This is because many surgeons believe new techniques of body contouring have made liposuction safer and that they generally offer better results. In contrast to society as a whole, health- and appearance-conscious individuals are giving themselves a wider variety of opportunities to excel in society by adopting healthier lifestyles. We are eating better, smoking and drinking less, and exercising more. We have learned that these are the keys to helping ourselves maintain both physical and mental health.

Although each of us possesses a unique size and shape, our bodies tend to respond differently to dieting and exercise. In many instances, we need only look at our parents to see what lies in store for our own bodies. Wide hips, small breasts, or sagging buttocks might be part of our genetic makeup and thus difficult to improve without surgical intervention. This is where body-contouring surgery can qualify as a gift you give yourself. There is little reason to ignore contour deformities when surgical sculpting techniques can improve or eliminate them.

Who is a candidate for body sculpting? Anyone, of any gender, who is in good health and is displeased with their present shape. Most patients who seek body contouring have struggled for years to improve their figures by dieting and exercise but have found that most of their faults can be only partially corrected with these measures.

Liposuction is not intended to remove massive amounts of fat; rather, it is designed to remove localized deposits of fat that are resistant to diet and exercise. In liposuction, fat is removed with a slender, hollow instrument called a cannula. This tubular instrument is inserted through a very small, well-hidden incision and attached to a suction machine, which literally vacuums fat from your body.

The body areas most commonly sculpted with liposuction are the thighs, abdomen, lower back (the location of "love handles" or "saddlebags"), and neck. In fact, any area of the body that harbors excess fat can be suctioned, including the face, arms, breasts, buttocks, or knees. However, liposuction is not recommended for the fat pads around the eyes. For these areas, surgical excision under direct vision is the treatment of choice.

The reason fat accumulates in the hips, thighs, buttocks, and abdomen is that fat in these areas is governed by the female hormone, estrogen. These fat deposits are there to provide extra energy during pregnancy and breastfeeding. Individuals with excess fat in these areas that does not respond to intelligent dieting and exercise are the ideal candidates for body-contouring liposuction. However, if you are overweight and see liposuction as a cure to obesity because you've found in the past that were not able to stick to a diet or exercise program, you are seeking the wrong solution. Liposuction *by itself* is not recommended! Rather, you should consult with nutritional and fitness professionals. If you believe that you might be addicted to food, you might seek the advice of an additional kind of professional: an addiction therapist. As I have previously stated, seeking counsel for the right reason is not a sign of weakness. Rather, it is a sign that you have come to grips with the fact that you have a problem and are resolved to becoming—and remaining—the person of your dreams. If you are truly committed to having a healthier and more attractive body, give yourself access to the wisdom and techniques that only a team of specialists can provide.

The woman whose before and after photographs are included below underwent an abdominoplasty (tummy tuck) along with liposuction of her lower back, hips, and thighs following a weight loss of one hundred pounds.

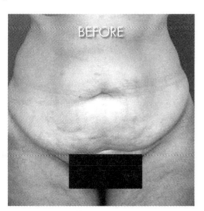 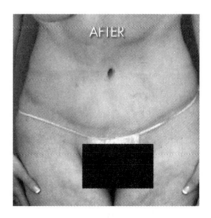

As demonstrated in this patient, a combination of intelligent weight loss and body-sculpting surgery can result in quite remarkable improvement. In her case, not only was her appearance and health enhanced but so was her self-image.

The following are facts that body-sculpting candidates should consider prior to embarking upon any enhancement program.

- Surgical sculpting procedures can be performed on most areas of your body.
- Your own postsurgical result will depend upon a number of variables, some of which are not under the control of your surgeon. They include your particular contour problems, your overall shape, your personalized surgical correction, and your compliance with the recommended dietary, nutritional, and exercise programs on a consistent and ongoing basis.

If you are considering body-contouring surgery, two other questions are relevant. First: Is it safe? Generally speaking, the answer is a resounding yes; however, it is surgery, and the risks that apply to all forms of surgery must be considered. As is the case with any surgery, your results are more likely to meet your expectations when the procedures are performed by skillful and experienced surgeons.

The second question is: Does it last? As was discussed in the sections on facial rejuvenation, the results of body-contouring surgery can be considered permanent in that the excess skin and fat are removed and discarded at the time of surgery. Even so, the aging process marches ever onward, and the need for further surgery to correct *new* sagging might arise as your biological clock continues to tick.

The Skin Factor

Healthy skin is also important when considering any body-enhancing procedure. That's why I dedicate a large part of this book to skin. If your skin still has good elasticity, your excess skin will shrink to fit your newly created form below once the bulges and bags have been removed and a new, thinner contour achieved. However, if your skin has not been cared for well and lacks elasticity, it will sag and form irregular contours, which might require surgical excision.

Healthy skin is a product of smart nutrition, protection from the damaging rays of the sun, and intelligent care—lifestyle choices addressed in other sections of this book. In addition to protection from excessive sun damage, you should adhere to moderation in drinking alcoholic beverages and in using nicotine-containing substances. Skin tone is also a reflection of how well you are aging. However, loose, sagging skin can occur anywhere in the body and at any age, especially in individuals who repeatedly lose and gain large amounts of weight.

Your overall body health or "biological age" seems to play an equally important role in how quickly—and well—you will heal from body-sculpting surgery. Most people return to work within three to five days and to normal activity within three weeks. Often, compression (girdle-like) garments are recommended.

As a rule, compression garments are provided by your surgeon. These garments provide support, reduce discomfort, and help the operated-upon areas to smoothly redrape the overlying skin. They also help prevent accumulation of serum or blood under the skin. Garments are usually worn for as long as three weeks and are easily hidden under your clothing.

One question often asked is, "Will the fat return if I gain weight?" Our bodies contain only a certain number of fat cells; therefore, if a surgeon removes some of these cells, the discarded ones cannot return. However, those that remain behind—and it is critical that some are left behind—can accumulate the oils that cause fat cells to expand. Following liposuction, significant weight gain will result in generalized obesity, but the gain seen within the suctioned areas will be less than in other parts of the body.

The Tummy Tuck Operation (Abdominoplasty)

Abdominoplasty, or the "tummy tuck," is a plastic surgical procedure designed to improve your waistline and lower abdomen by addressing the weakening muscles and excess skin and fat of your abdomen. Like liposuction, abdominoplasty is neither a shortcut to nor a substitute for weight loss and generally is most successful in those men and women who do not exhibit generalized obesity. The best results are obtained in patients who exhibit localized areas of excess abdominal skin and fat and who abide by good nutritional and fitness habits.

A waistline that does not respond to weight loss, exercise, and muscle toning is often compounded by an anatomical defect in the abdominal wall—a hernia of sorts. Rather than remaining attached to each other, the two main muscles in the abdomen (the rectus abdominis) become separated, allowing the intestines to push against the thinner sheet of muscle covering them and cause it to protrude outward. Therefore, these muscles must be reattached in order to produce a stronger abdominal wall.

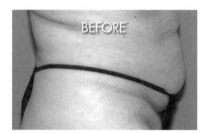 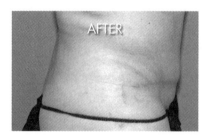

Photos courtesy of Dr. Brentley Taylor.

If, however, you have only a mild excess of skin, localized fat, and no muscle laxity, a suction lipectomy (liposuction) might be all that is indicated.

Convalescence from abdominoplasty usually takes four to six weeks, during which time the abdomen might feel tight, requiring you to restrict activities and wear loose clothing.

Occasionally, certain fat deposits on the sides of the abdomen become more noticeable after abdominoplasty and must be removed with a second touch-up operation, which can usually be performed under local anesthesia. Although abdominoplasty is one of the more extensive cosmetic procedures undertaken, the improvements in certain figure faults can be dramatic, providing an overall improvement in the shape of your body.

Hopefully, the information provided in this book will provide insight into surgical and nonsurgical body contouring as well as facial and nasal surgery. Through my own experience along with contributions over the years from colleagues who have specialized in body-contouring procedures, my intent is to dispel many of the myths concerning appearance-enhancing procedures and products and to provide you with the information you need to make wise decisions as you move toward becoming the person of your dreams. The next few chapters reveal additional procedures and measures that could help you reach that goal.

CHAPTER 31

The Male Factor

When I launched my facial plastic surgery practice, only about 5 percent of the patients undergoing appearance-enhancing surgery at that time were men. Today, men make up approximately a third of the patients who consult with me. The natural response to this evolutionary demographic is to ask, Why are more men now open to undergoing elective procedures designed to help them appear younger and more attractive? The answer is driven as much by economics as by what a less informed segment of our society might consider vanity.

Let's explore the factor of vanity. In my opinion, to be vain is to be so obsessed with your appearance that it interferes with your ability to function effectively in society. To exhibit pride in your appearance, however, is to honor the "temple of your soul"—your body. The more I think about the purpose of our bodies, the more inclined I am to look upon them as biological incubators, cauldrons that house our souls while they are being put to the test.

Since 1975, the job market has changed dramatically. It is no secret that more women are being hired for jobs that were once primarily available to men. Also, more males have come to realize what women learned centuries ago: in any competitive marketplace, looks matter. A youthful appearance matters. First impressions matter. They matter in being hired, in being promoted, in extending your career, and when attempting to attract a companion or mate. Most of all, they matter in your impression of yourself. As a popular Whitney Houston song correctly told us, the greatest love of all is learning to love yourself.

I once helped a legendary college football coach—whose name and face were easily recognizable to the masses—appear younger in person, when photographed, and in front of television cameras. He was very much aware of the effect his presence had on others. As the coach's face began to show the results of aging and of years of being exposed to the elements, he shared with me that young recruits and their families were beginning to ask how much longer he planned to coach. This high-profile coach became convinced that retirement was imminent simply because he was looking old enough to retire. He recognized what recruits and their families had already recognized: his aging appearance hampered his ability to lure the level of talent upon which he had built his championship reputation. In addition to the coach's own analysis of his condition, his agent boldly informed the coach that he "looked old" on television and in the commercials that contributed to a significant part of the coach's income. So, for his career and the related economic reasons, the coach decided to do something about his aging appearance. He asked me to perform a facial procedure that helped him look ten years younger. In return, the surgery helped him become a more effective recruiter during the final years of his career and an even more effective spokesperson for the companies for whom he performed commercials.

Then there was the case of a celebrity movie and television actor who consulted with me about performing rejuvenation surgery upon him. He had noticed that his career as an actor appeared to be winding down. He also shared that he had undergone a facelift and eyelid surgery some years back and had seen a surge in his career shortly thereafter. However, as the signs of advancing age began to creep in once more, the roles to which he had become accustomed were becoming fewer and farther between. After I performed a combination of facial rejuvenation procedures on him, the actor was asked to join the cast of a popular Western television series. Shortly thereafter, he was given the starring role in another series.

These are just two examples of men who benefitted from appearance-enhancing surgery. I could cite numerous others, including the CEO of one of the world's top telecommunications companies, television anchors, news correspondents, politicians, and educators. All were able to extend their careers by having "some work done," as appearance enhancement is referred to in such circles.

As an appearance-enhancement physician and surgeon, I witness similar stories on a daily basis. I could also share countless other cases in which a man's lifestyle changes and attention to his appearance not only improved his outward appearance but restored his self-esteem and, in many cases, led him to become more conscious of his health. Each of these factors allowed these men to become more competitive for a longer time in whatever marketplaces they chose to compete, including matters of the heart.

As occurs in women, and regardless of our outward appearance, we men also see a reduction in the levels of our sex hormone as the years pass by. Our circulating levels of testosterone, the male sex hormone, slowly but steadily begin to diminish beginning in our late thirties. Because the reduction in testosterone does not occur rapidly, we do not usually experience the physical and mental changes that often accompany menopause in women. In men, the condition is known as andropause. Scientific testing and professional regulation of a man's hormones can often restore muscle mass, energy levels, and libido, thus improving our self-image and the overall quality of our lives.

To further enhance a man's appeal index—and thus his career—some men might also require mind/body counseling, including coaching on wardrobe, hairstyle, posture, weight management, dentition, and behavioral patterns. However, not until some major life event occurs do most men come to this realization. In addition to career-ending threats, a large majority of the men I see in my practice have lost a mate, either though divorce or death. Prior to those events, they became complacent—and, frankly, more than a bit careless—about paying attention to their appeal index. The truth is that it takes more than a hair transplant or the removal of drooping and baggy skin and fat around the eyes and underneath the chin to help these male patients become their personal best again. It takes a comprehensive evaluation of all the factors that have been neglected over the years and a personalized treatment plan designed to create a younger, more fit, and more natural-appearing version of the person these men were in their prime—in some cases, the person of their dreams. That's why a prospective patient—male or female—should consult an appearance-enhancement surgeon who is connected with professionals qualified to address all the factors needed to give their patients the knowledge, service, and encouragement needed to recapture many of the attributes that existed during their youthful years.

The man whose before and after photographs are included below underwent facial rejuvenation surgery. His case was somewhat unusual in that he was already familiar with the other rejuvenation initiatives addressed throughout this book. He had come up through the marketing and advertising industry and was more than familiar with how the way a person looks tends to define who they are.

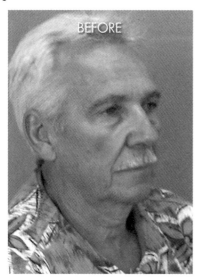
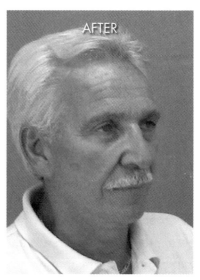

I continue to stay in touch with this former patient, who chose to participate in an ultimate makeover television production aired by an ABC affiliate in Pensacola, Florida. Nearly fifteen years following his surgery, he continues to look much younger than men his own age.

One of the factors that tend to cause men to shy away from appearance-enhancing surgery is the eerie way some entertainers and high-profile men look following plastic surgery. Some barely resemble themselves and have thus seen their careers plummet rather than be vaulted forward. Remember: it is not *undergoing* plastic surgery that determines whether a natural appearance is achieved or whether one is left with an unnatural appearance; it is *how the surgery is performed*—and by whom.

That's why, throughout this book, I recommend ways to find a surgeon that will provide what men want and need—a naturally more youthful appearance.

Although the high-profile men I've assisted, helping them to extend their careers and become more appealing potential mates, often appeared on television, in the movies, or in print, I strongly doubt that you or anyone you know suspected that they had undergone facial surgery. The reason is rather basic: like my elite appearance-enhancing colleagues, I choose to take an approach not always practiced in the highly competitive centers identified with cosmetic surgery. In men, I usually recommend a graduated approach to the appearance-enhancement process, especially in the facial areas. In addition, I study their earlier photographs to determine how their faces appeared before the advanced signs of aging began to set in. Only then do I design the treatment plan I intend to carry out in order to restore their more youthful appearances.

An appearance-altering professional must refrain from creating a *different* face, especially in a high-profile male patient. Something that is not well known outside plastic surgery circles is that, some years ago, a procedure designed to convert an upper eyelid common to Asian populations into an upper lid that appears more occidental (Western) found its way into the male plastic surgery arena. When performed on a Caucasian man, the technique significantly alters the appearance around the eye area—in my opinion, to the extreme. Many of the male entertainers who exhibit what is often referred to as the "plastic look" likely had this upper eyelid technique performed by a colleague that did not follow the advice and opinions on this subject that I offer in this book, in lectures, in peer-reviewed articles, and in textbooks.

One in particular comes to mind. This highly recognizable entertainer consulted me for appearance-enhancing surgery. He had already consulted with other surgeons who recommended procedures I advised against. This man chose not to follow my recommendations and to instead go with the recommendations offered by another surgeon. His appearance was changed to the extreme—so much so that he has become, in the appearance-altering industry, the example that the men and women who consult with me say they want to avoid.

Not only men but anyone contemplating appearance-altering surgery should inquire as to which techniques the surgeon intends to use and what they are intended to achieve. Keep in mind that there is no one-size-fits-all approach to enhancing a person's appearance.

As your own best advocate (one of the gifts you give yourself), I recommend that you request to see before and after photographs of patients who have undergone treatment by that surgeon for the same or similar conditions as you so that you can be assured that techniques that will produce an appearance that fits your gender, nationality, and wishes will be used in your case. In short, take nothing for granted!

It is often overlooked that from his shoulders up, a well-groomed man looks the same from morning to night, whether he is wearing a T-shirt or tuxedo. Women, on the other hand, change their appearance for the circumstances at hand. The hairstyle and makeup a woman wears during the day might differ from the one she wears when she dresses for a formal affair or special event. The bottom line is that friends and associates are accustomed to seeing women's appearances change. We are not accustomed to seeing the same degree of change occur among men.

With that thought in mind, elite appearance-enhancing specialists avoid drastic changes in a man's appearance. Smaller steps, rather than giant leaps, are often the best practice. The best appearance-enhancing results are obtained when friends and colleagues comment, "Have you lost weight?" or "You look great. There's something different about you. What is it?"

Following appearance-enhancing surgery, some men allow their hair to grow a bit longer. Some blend away a hint of gray. Some grow a mustache or beard for a while, just so they can respond to inquiries with, "I have been focusing on my weight. I have been exercising more and getting more rest—and what do you think about my new hairstyle (or beard)?"

In most cases, that is enough of a distraction to deflect the observer's attention away from the fact that appearance-enhancing surgery was performed.

But a man's rejuvenated appearance requires more than a younger-looking face, less droopy eyelids, or a more youthful, straighter nose. It requires attention to the other things addressed throughout this book: posture, wardrobe, a positive attitude, weight management, skin care—all the things that create an aura around a man that make people of all ages and genders want to be in his presence and proudly introduce him as their friend, mate, or associate.

While it is true that high-profile men comprise a significant segment of those men who choose to give themselves the gift of looking and feeling their best, we tend to overlook the fact that the vast majority of appearance-enhancing procedures are performed on the men who make the wheels of society run more smoothly *outside* the limelight. In my own practice, I help men in the military services, educators, business owners, entrepreneurs, law enforcement, and all manner of sales professionals maintain—or regain—a more competitive appearance.

A few years back, I received the following letter from a grateful male patient who had been involved in an accident during which he sustained multiple injuries to his face and nose. As I corrected the conditions resulting from his accident, I also included many of the life-enhancement factors addressed in this chapter and throughout this book.

This man's business dealt primarily with buying and selling cars and trucks. This is part of the letter he sent to me:

> *Dear Dr. McCollough,*
> *The surgery you performed on me has truly had a positive influence on my life. As I have said on many occasions: "face to riches . . ."*
>
> *The positives in my life are enormous. I can breathe better, resulting in more restful sleep. My business is up, while others are complaining theirs is down. I am receiving compliments on my eyes, and looks are coming my way again, installing confidence, and yes, I've met a really great lady.*
>
> *As you assured me (prior to performing my surgery), my face is not perfect; but it is a better face.*

I just wanted to take time to thank you and your team for helping make all this possible.

Sincerely,

E. L.

In my experience, this man's story is the rule rather than the exception. I also appreciate his mentioning my staff in his letter. Helping someone who previously felt as though his future had permanently been altered in a negative manner as a result of an accident is, indeed, a team effort. Not only must the surgeon restore the patient's features as closely as possible to their appearance before the event; their team of like-minded professionals must also provide the necessary psychological support to set the patient's mind right as they reenter the multifaceted world of competition.

This story presented above also underscores the necessary relationship, in the life-enhancement package, between the health aspect (more restful sleep) and how an enhanced self-image translates to success in business and in matters of the heart. I offer it here as yet another example of how appearance- and life-enhancing professionals—with the cooperation of an informed, willing, and compliant patient—can achieve outcomes that are unachievable unless a mutually trusting doctor-patient relationship is established at the outset of treatment.

Because hair loss is most often identified with men, the next chapter addresses this troublesome—yet increasingly correctable—condition.

CHAPTER 32

The Hair Factor

During my quest to become an appearance-enhancing surgeon, I learned that there was a way to correct a dreaded phenomenon in men and women: hair loss. Upon this realization, I sought out the most revered hair transplantation surgeons in the field. I made a list and set out to learn as much as possible from the best of the best.

My first stop was Beverly Hills, California, where I studied with Dr. Charles Monell (the partner of Dr. Walter Berman). Then it was on to Boston, Massachusetts, where I studied with Dr. Richard Webster. Next, I traveled to Hot Springs, Arkansas, to learn the techniques of Dr. Bluford Stough and finally to New York City, where a lasting friendship with Dr. Norman Orentreich began. Among other well-deserved accolades, Dr. Orentreich is known as the "father of hair replacement surgery." He discovered the breakthrough procedure that has allowed millions of men and women who've lost hair on one part of their head to have it replaced with hair taken from the scalp on the sides and back. Norman proved that hair follicles (roots) taken from those regions would grow wherever in the body they were transplanted, including areas of the scalp that had gone bald. He also discovered the cause of baldness in men and women. It is hormonal in nature, related to the conversion of the male hormone, testosterone, to a form that could be excreted through our kidneys; yet until dihydrotestosterone is excreted, the end product of testosterone reeks havoc on the predisposed follicles at the front and on top of the scalp in men and women whose genetic code renders them susceptible to male-pattern baldness.

At the completion of my training, I proudly brought the science and craft I learned from these pioneers in hair restoration surgery back with me to UAB's medical center in Birmingham, Alabama, where I shared the knowledge and techniques I had learned with the staff and students and began to perform hair transplantation and other forms of hair restoration surgery in my own practice.

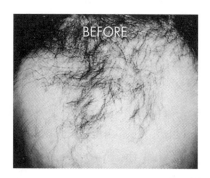 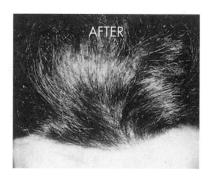

An example of hair restoration surgery.

A few years later, I handed off that portion of my practice to a younger associate. Since that time, the surgical techniques have improved, including transferring large flaps of scalp from the sides of the head to the frontal hairline areas. Another technique minimizes the area of baldness on the top of the head by serially removing and discarding portions of scalp in that region that do not bear hair and advancing the hairline upward from the sides toward the top, thus reducing the number of grafted hairs required to provide coverage.

Based upon Dr. Orentreich's research, medical science has discovered ways to help prevent baldness in some patients. The hard truth is that just as hairstyles come and go, so does the hair that exists on our heads. Most of us will experience some degree of hair loss during our lifetime. This opens the door for profit-driven individuals and companies to propagate all manner of products and devices that claim to correct baldness. Once again, the "buyer beware" admonition holds true. I strongly recommend that you check with your dermatologist or hair restoration surgeon before purchasing a baldness remedy from a television ad.

To assist you in your research, in this section I focus on scientific explanations for conditions that impact a person's appearance, health, and well-being, including their self-esteem. If you are beginning to see the hair on your head thin, I also provide ways that you can give yourself access to scientifically tested remedies designed to eliminate or improve upon the condition, including platelet rich plasma (PRP). This treatment involves drawing a vial of blood, which is spun down and the nutrient-rich plasma injected into your scalp. Since being reported by a Japanese scientist in 2011, the process has been shown to stimulate new hair growth as a result of a thickened epithelium of the hair follicle as well as an increase in the number of collagen fibers and blood vessels.[9] To learn more, research on the internet or contact one of the hair and skin specialists at my clinic by visiting McColloughPlasticSurgery.com.

You might also be one of the millions of people who are dealing with unwanted hair growth in various areas of your body. If so, you might be experiencing the kind of hormonal imbalances that accompany the aging process.

The most common type of hair loss on the top and sides of the head is known as male-pattern baldness, or androgenic alopecia. Because both men and women have androgenic (male) hormones in their bodies, this condition occurs in both genders and commonly creates embarrassment. If so, you have several choices. You can camouflage the areas of thinning or baldness with artificial hair or attempt to revive sickly hair follicles with medications, hormone therapy, or injections of your own plasma, as suggested above. If these measures fail, you might want to consult a hair transplantation surgeon who can replace thinning areas with individual hair grafts taken from the back and sides of your scalp.

Hereditary male-pattern baldness is the most common kind of hair loss. In genetically susceptible individuals, certain sex hormones (testosterone and, to a lesser extent, cortisol) trigger a particular pattern of permanent hair loss. In men, this type of hair thinning occurs in the temple areas of the scalp and can begin as early as puberty.

In my practice, I have seen hormonal imbalances cause temporary hair loss. The most common cause is abnormally low levels of thyroid hormones, as well as the hormonal swings that occur with pregnancy, childbirth, sudden discontinuation of birth control pills, or the onset of menopause (in women) or andropause (in men).

---

9. M. Takikawa et al, "Enhanced effect of platelet-rich plasma containing a new carrier on hair growth," Dermatologic Survey 37, no. 12 (December 2011): 1721–9, https://doi.org/10.1111/j.1524-4725.2011.02123.x.

The key factor is whether the hair follicle (root) is merely traumatized or has been irrevocably damaged. Let's examine some of the conditions that can cause your hair to thin, break off, or fall out.

- **Thyroid imbalances:** Your thyroid gland helps regulate hormone levels in your body. If the gland isn't working properly, hair loss can result.
- **Alopecia areata:** This condition occurs when your body's immune system suddenly attacks hair follicles, causing smooth, roundish patches of hair loss scattered over your scalp. In most cases, the hair returns to areas of baldness, only to recur at unexpected times.
- **Scalp infections:** Infections (ringworm, for example) can invade the hair and skin of your scalp, leading to hair loss. Once these types of infections are treated, lost hair generally grows back.
- **Other skin disorders:** Diseases that can cause scarring (such as lichen planus and some types of lupus) can result in permanent hair loss, especially in areas where the scarring occurred.

Hair loss can also be caused by drugs used to treat cancer, arthritis, depression, heart problems, and high blood pressure. Other factors include the following.

- **Traumatic alopecia:** Many people experience a general thinning of hair several months after a physical or emotional shock. Examples include sudden or excessive weight loss, a high fever, or a catastrophic event in one's life. Direct trauma to the scalp, such as pressure applied by tightly fitting head dressings, bumping one's head on a cabinet door, surgical incisions, or being struck with a blunt object, can also cause this type of hair loss.
- **Hair-pulling disorder:** Also known as "traction alopecia," this emotionally based illness causes people to have an irresistible urge to pull out their hair, whether it's from the scalp, their eyebrows, or other areas of the body. Traction on hair shafts often leaves patchy bald spots

on the head. However, because the roots (follicles) are rarely damaged, the hair will grow back if hair-pulling ceases.

- **Hairstyle alopecia:** This is a term I originated, and it is another form of hair-pulling alopecia. It a form of traction alopecia, but is not intentionally generated. Hairstyle alopecia can occur when the hair is pulled too tightly with any form of hair styling, the most common being tightly pulled ponytails. However, pigtails or cornrows can also create this condition. Anytime the hair is tightly and consistently pulled (regardless of the direction), the hair shafts will become up-rooted from their follicles, leading to thinning or baldness. Because, in hairstyle alopecia, the roots/follicles themselves are not damaged, this condition, too, usually subsides once the offending behavior is eliminated . . . unless other factors addressed in this book come into play.

- **Genetic alopecia:** Your risk of hair loss increases if relatives on either side of your family experienced hair loss. Your genetic code (or genome) also affects the age at which you might begin to lose hair and the developmental speed, pattern, and extent of the baldness experienced.

- **Hair treatments:** Overuse or improper use of certain offending chemicals, such as hair-coloring products, hair-straightening products, and permanent waves, can leave your hair brittle and prone to breaking off at the level of the scalp. Once again, as long as the roots (follicles) are not overly traumatized, hair will continue to grow from them. A good example of this principle exists in the horticultural world. Many plants are pruned each season. As the coming months ensue, new growth originates from the pruned areas. With respect to chemical "pruning agents," once these products and practices are eliminated from one's lifestyle routines, the issue of brittleness should subside.

- **Poor nutrition:** Hair density might become thinner when you skimp on good dietary sources of iron and protein, such as red meat, nonfat dairy products, and iron-fortified cereal. Hair loss related to poor nutrition often accompanies starvation eating disorders (such as anorexia) and crash dieting, both of which are conditions individuals give

238 | The Gift You Give Yourself

to themselves. The good news is that this kind of hair loss is correctable when the perpetrators give themselves the green light to reverse the conditions they created.

Medical Treatment of Hair Loss

While a plethora of products claim to prevent and restore hair loss, much of this is hype. A few medical products on the market have been shown to prevent hair loss. One of them is the liquid form of a drug known as minoxidil, marketed under the trade name Rogaine. The topical application of this drug is helpful in minimizing early male-pattern baldness, which can be exacerbated by testosterone replacement therapy. The off-setting drug to this process (and treatment program) is finasteride. It was originally used to treat benign enlargement of the prostate gland in men. It works by preventing the final metabolic conversion of testosterone to dihydrotestosterone, the product that—once it is taken by your blood-stream to susceptible areas containing hair follicles—actually poisons hair follicles. The follicles on top of your head are the most susceptible. Those that occupy areas of your scalp along the sides and back tend to resist the process. Thus, follicles taken from those regions and transplanted to the top of the scalp are used during hair restoration surgery. This discovery was made by my friend Dr. Norman Orentreich, who, during his career, was one of the world's most elite dermatologists and age-management research advocates.

Minoxidil (Rogaine) is a drug originally designed to treat high blood pressure. When taken orally, the medication causes blood vessels all over the body to dilate, thereby decreasing blood pressure. This process appears to be beneficial to hair follicles subject to the poisonous effects of dihydrotestosterone in susceptible men and women.

Scientific tests and clinical observations have shown both drugs (minoxidil and finasteride) and PRP injections to be effective in treating male-pattern baldness. Before initiating a course of treatment, you should investigate other factors. Hypothyroidism (lower than optimal levels of thyroid hormone) is a common condition that affects many men and women. Simple blood tests can determine whether this factor is contributing to your hair loss.

As is the case with most "medical discoveries," these treatments for hair loss were discovered while some other condition was being investigated. Orentreich was researching causes of the skin condition psoriasis. In some of the patients taking minoxidil to treat their high blood pressure, an unusual side effect was noticed. Some who had been losing their hair began to experience new hair growth. As a result, clinical studies were begun using minoxidil applied topically to the scalp. My good friend and fellow author Andy Andrews described this phenomenon in his best-selling book *The Noticer*. It is based upon comments passed on to him by a mentor—a man he knew only as "Jones." When asked how he knew about so many things, Jones replied, "I notice things that other people overlook . . . I notice things about situations and people that produce perspective. So I give them that broader view . . . and it allows them to regroup, take a breath, and begin their lives again."[10] Although I did not realize it when *The Noticer* was published, I had been noticing for as long as I can remember. I still am. I hope you will join the legions of "noticers" who are giving themselves the best chance to learn from the giants who preceded them, and I hope that you can, if called for, begin your life again. Apply those lessons to modern-day conditions and circumstances, and then excel in an increasingly complex world.

It appears that minoxidil stimulates existing follicles to grow longer, coarser hairs, though at time of writing, medical experts are still unsure of the exact mechanism involved. It does not stimulate the growth of new follicles or revive those in which activity no longer exists. Strangely enough, drugs used to treat cancer (chemotherapy drugs) tend to affect struggling hair follicles in a positive way. Following a course of chemotherapy, the hair in areas not susceptible to male-pattern baldness not only comes back but does so thicker, wavier, and curlier. I have witnessed

10. Andy Andrews, *The Noticer* (Nashville: Thomas Nelson, 2009).

this phenomenon in patients for whom I personally performed hair transplantation surgery. Hair follicles successfully transplanted into balding areas grew thicker, wavier hair that provided greater coverage than the hair shafts prior to chemotherapy treatment.

Minoxidil is applied topically to balding or thinning areas of the scalp twice a day. It is a clear, colorless, odorless liquid that can be either sprayed or rubbed on the scalp. While two-thirds of patients using minoxidil experience new hair growth, one-third obtain minimal, if any, results and continue to lose their hair. Whether these patients were tested for other conditions that cause hair loss (such as thyroid or sex hormone imbalances) is not known.

Some patients treated with minoxidil notice that hair loss slows down, but their bald areas remain the same. Others notice some improvement in their balding pattern. This improvement is confined to the top of the head, as, unfortunately, minoxidil does not appear to influence frontal balding (i.e., male-pattern baldness) in any patients—male or female. For yet unexplained reasons, minoxidil appears to be more affective in women than in men. As an avowed "noticer," I can only speculate that further studies on the contributions of estrogen and testosterone must take place.

In order to determine its effectiveness in any given user, minoxidil must be used continuously for at least three to six months. A fact little publicized by the pharmaceutical industry is that it is necessary to continue using the drug indefinitely in order to maintain any beneficial results that might be experienced. If you begin to use minoxidil and then stop, expect to see hair that was prevented from falling out do so rather rapidly. Your hair loss pattern will revert to that which existed prior to beginning therapy. The bottom line is that minoxidil is merely a treatment for hair loss, not the long-sought cure.

Unexplained Autoimmune Hair Loss

Alopecia areata most commonly occurs in people younger than twenty, but children and adults of any age can be affected. Women and men are affected equally.

Alopecia areata is suspected when clumps of hair fall out in areas of the scalp that were previously covered with hair, resulting in totally smooth, rounded patches of hairlessness. In some cases, the hair may become thinner, without noticeable patches of baldness, or it may grow and then suddenly break off, leaving short stubs (called "exclamation point" stubble). In rare cases, complete loss of scalp hair and body hair occurs. Hair loss associated with alopecia areata often comes and goes within a period of months, but hair may fall out in another region of the scalp. Although the new hair is usually the same color and texture as the rest of the hair, it sometimes returns finer and whiter. Unfortunately, this phenomenon does not appear to affect unwanted hair growth in other areas of the body.

About 10 percent of people with this condition never regrow hair. Individuals who are more likely to experience permanent hair loss include those who:

- Have a family history of the condition.
- Have the condition at a young age (before puberty) or for longer than one year.
- Are troubled by another autoimmune disease.
- Are prone to allergies.
- Have extensive hair loss as a result of the condition.
- Have abnormal color, shape, texture, or thickness of the fingernails or toenails.

Because hair is a product of the same "stem cells" that produce skin and nails and because your hair is an important part of your appearance, hair loss can result in feeling unattractive and loss of self-esteem. Some people who experience alopecia areata find that their fingernails and toenails become pitted, as if a pin or needle had made many tiny dents in them. They might also take on the appearance of sandpaper.

Although alopecia areata cannot be "cured," it can be treated. I recommend consultation with a dermatologist who specializes in hair loss and restoration, because most people who experience one episode will experience more.

Hormonal Causes of Hair Loss

The condition known as hypothyroidism is characterized by a collection of symptoms, including weight gain, facial puffiness, extremity edema, dry skin, fatigue, constipation, and hair loss.

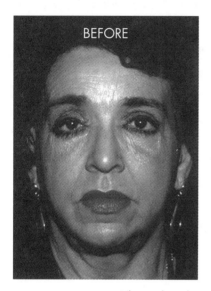
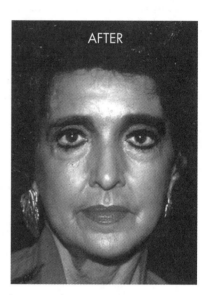

Thyroid replacement therapy alone.

It is easy to test for thyroid hormone deficiency. Even if tests indicate that hormone levels are "within normal limits," you could be one of those patients with "normal" laboratory values who still exhibits one or more symptoms of thyroid deficiency. If so, you could benefit from empirical (that is, "treat the patient rather than the lab results") thyroid replacement therapy. This is an application of clinical medicine I learned from Dr. Tinsley R. Harrison, the metaphysician who literally wrote the textbook that today's doctors still study in medical school and beyond.

Just because a laboratory result indicates that a life-sustaining element is within the "normal" range does not mean that it is within the *optimal* range, where the amount needed for the body owner to perform at an exceptional level is present. As is the case with most laboratory values, the individual generally feels, looks, and performs better if the values are elevated to the optimal levels, above the 50 percent range of normal. The best example I can give to emphasize this is exhibited in the gasoline industry. When you pull up to the pump at a gas station, you possess the gift to choose between a low-grade, medium-grade, or high-grade fuel. The low-grade fuel barely meets the standards required by most vehicles. The high-grade fuel is created to meet the requirements of high-performance vehicles. The same can be said about the human body. If you, as a body owner, are willing to accept the bare minimum indicators, you can never expect to perform at maximum potential. I can think of no greater reason for all body owners to commit to giving themselves the best opportunity to perform at maximum potential in a complex and highly competitive world. This kind of insight can only be obtained through scientific testing, whether the condition in question is hair loss or total body health.

Your body, the incubator of your soul, was created with the ability to balance imbalances—up to a point. However, as a body owner, you are expected to do your part in the ongoing creation process and contribute to the initiative.

In females, reduction in female sex hormones (estrogen) and a relative increase in the male hormone (testosterone) occur during menopause. This causes hairs on the head to begin to fall out in patients who are genetically prone to developing male-pattern baldness. Testosterone is produced by both the testicles and the adrenal glands. In males, testosterone levels are—by design—the dominant gender hormone, but all men also produce small levels of estrogen. On the other hand, estrogen is the predominant hormone in females, but women—at all ages—also produce small amounts of testosterone.

In both genders, these hormones are eventually broken down by a complex metabolic process into a form that can be excreted through the urinary tract. The aforementioned Dr. Norman Orentreich was the first to recognize that the final product of testosterone metabolism, dihydrotestosterone, is poisonous to hair follicles that are genetically predisposed to die when they come into contact with circulating levels of dihydrotestosterone in the bloodstream, which raises the question: Does increasing the circulation of dihydrotestosterone-carrying blood to areas of the scalp that contain susceptible hair follicles create a favorable or unfavorable set of circumstances? Perhaps, with further research, the answer will be forthcoming sooner rather than later.

In women, menopause marks the sudden tapering of circulating estrogens. As estrogen levels drop, the small amount of testosterone in a woman's system begins to result in powerful clinical manifestations, including hair loss in the scalp, growth of facial hair, lowering of the pitch of the voice, and reduction in breast fullness.

A trained health-care professional or total health spa can test for all hormone levels and return them to balance by prescribing a gamut of replacement alternatives. In many cases, hair loss can be stabilized before it progresses to a state of baldness, thereby eliminating the current trend of styling that includes men shaving their heads or women wearing wigs.

Surgical Correction of Baldness

Because hair styling is recognized as an appearance-enhancing and first-impression factor, hair loss is one of the most frustrating conditions a person can experience. The best time to begin hair transplantation is when the frontal hairline first begins to recede. Hair transplantation can also camouflage additional hair loss, if and when it occurs.

Since the introduction of the hair transplant in the 1950s by the afore-mentioned Dr. Norman Orentreich, techniques for hair replacement have been refined, and the number of different procedures has grown enor-mously. Surgery that can now be offered to patients includes standard hair transplant "plugs," minigraft plugs, micrografts, hairline advancements (scalp reduction), extensive scalp lifting, and flap-transposition opera-tions. These procedures can be used independently or in combination to fit each individual hair loss pattern.

Who Should Have Hair Replacement Surgery?

Patients present for hair replacement with varying degrees of baldness. If you are completely bald on the top of your head with only a thin rim of hair around the back from ear to ear, surgeons may advise against surgical hair replacement. In such cases, the area to be covered may be too large for the amount of donor hair available. Hairline advancement surgery (scalp reduction) may allow you to become a candidate for hair transplantation. If you are primarily bald along your frontal hairline, you may be a good candidate for a scalp transposition flap.

If your hairline has receded because it was surgically lifted as part of an ill-conceived facelift procedure, your hairline can be surgically lowered, either in the forehead region or behind the ears. Incisions for hairline-lowering procedures are created in such a way that the residual hair will grow through the scar, thereby making the incision site virtually invisible. In some cases, a hairline can be lowered as much as an inch with each procedure. Multiple procedures can be performed to create additional lowering; however, it is advisable to wait six to twelve months between procedures. Doing so allows the scalp to stretch so that the hairline can be moved downward. This same technique can be used to correct small areas of the scalp on which scarring has prevented hair growth. The scar can be removed and the edges of hair-bearing scalp brought together, thereby eliminating the area of scalp that does not bear hair.

Hairpieces that adhere to the scalp with the assistance of nonirritating glues are recommended in cases where surgery is not advisable. I don't believe anything artificial should be placed *into* the scalp to secure hairpieces. I have seen serious complications arise from doing so.

If you have thick, curly, or wavy hair and have a receding hairline, or a patch of baldness on the top of your scalp or crown, you are the ideal candidate for hair transplantation. If your hair is simply thinning, you may or may not be a candidate for hair replacement surgery. You might be a candidate for some of the medical therapies discussed in the previous chapter.

As you can see, each case is different and requires an individually programmed master plan by a hair replacement specialist.

Hair Transplantation Surgery

Hair transplantation is a surgical procedure that involves taking tiny grafts from the hair-bearing parts of the scalp on the back and sides of the head and moving them to the bald areas. Once the grafts are removed, graded, and cleaned, they are transplanted into the receptor sites in the bald areas. Minigrafts and individual hair grafts may be used to give a more soft and subtle look to the frontal hairline.

The procedure is designed to transplant the roots of the hair. Once the transplanted roots have established their new place of residence, they usually produce hairs for as long as they would have had they remained in the donor sites.

While some of the techniques for removing and transplanting hair follicles are new, hair transplantation surgery has been used for more than seventy years with highly successful results. Roots successfully transplanted years ago are still producing new hairs every few months.

The Procedure

In order to provide the thickest coverage to any given bald area, several procedures may be required.

With today's technology, the vast majority of transplanted hair follicles survive transplantation. This percentage is usually enough to provide an acceptable result when the procedure is carried to conclusion.

Micrografts

Unlike the grafts that were used for the first fifty years of hair transplantation surgery, micrografts are comprised of single hair follicle. These smaller grafts tend to give a more natural appearance to the frontal hairlines. The benefit of using smaller grafts is that there is less tufting because the grafts can be placed closer together per stage than standard grafts. Using smaller grafts, patient may require only two or three procedures rather than the four procedures that were standard with conventional grafts, which are about the size of the click at the top of a ballpoint pen and contain from four to six follicles. The size of grafts can be discussed with your surgeon at the time of consultation.

Once new hairs from the transplanted roots have reached the surface of the skin, they ordinarily grow at approximately half an inch per month.

It should be apparent, then, that from the day the first stage is performed, you—as a hair transplantation patient—must be willing to wait several months for the new hair to grow long enough to provide coverage of the bald or thinned areas. With each subsequent stage, the hair gets thicker and provides even better coverage.

Although the coverage provided by hair transplantation is never as thick as what existed prior to any hair loss, with proper styling, an uncomplicated case can usually obtain a satisfactory result and an enhanced self-image.

CHAPTER 33

The Lifelong Value of

Appearance Enhancement in Your Younger Years

Having established that the way we look has everything to do with if, when, and how wide the doors of opportunity swing open for us, it stands to reason that the earlier we start enhancing our looks, the more years we will have to reap the benefits of the best possible versions of ourselves.

This chapter reinforces the theme of early detection and prevention that permeates this book. As such, many of the procedures I address here are covered in more detail in other sections of this book. In this chapter, I address them as they apply specifically to young people. Depending upon your current age, they may apply to you, to your children, or to your grandchildren. If either of the latter applies, giving your child or grandchild the gift of enhancing their self-esteem could be one that alters their life in a positive way for a lifetime.

In chapter 15, I mentioned a patient in her early forties who consulted with me about performing an otoplasty on her. To protect her identify, we'll call her "Sally Jones." During Sally's consultation, she did share with me that she was afraid of general anesthesia and wanted to have the procedure performed with mild sedation and local anesthesia, but initially, she did not go into detail about why she wanted to have her protruding ears corrected. That would come later, during the middle of her surgery. It was then that I found out about an incident that took place when she was a preteen and that is the reason I'm including her story in this chapter.

At the conclusion of her consultation, we agreed upon the procedure and the date. While I was performing her operation, Sally began to cry. I immediately asked, "Am I hurting you?"

"No," she said.

I replied, "Can you tell me why you are crying?"

"Because I'm so happy," she answered.

So I laid down my instruments and said, "Tell me about it."

"When I was eleven years old," she began, "I went to a swimming party. When I got out of the pool, my hair was wet, and my large ears protruded right through. One of my classmates screamed so that everyone present could hear, 'My God, look at her ears!' From that time forward, I was known by my classmates as 'Ears Jones.'"

She went on, "I've not been swimming since I was eleven years old, but once we scheduled this surgery, I went to a department store and bought myself two bathing suits. I can't wait to go swimming with my new ears."

This patient's story is not that unusual in my practice. I often learn that embarrassing events that took place early in my patients' lives have had lasting effects, even into their advancing years.

So the question that you should ask is this: How young is too young to correct a feature that detracts from a person's appearance and self-esteem? My answer is a simple one: it depends.

In recent years, a nonsurgical procedure to correct irregularities in an infant's ears has gained popularity within pediatric and appearance-enhancing specialties. If the ears are splinted within the first few weeks of life, the externally applied splint will cause the underlying cartilage to assume the shape of the splint.

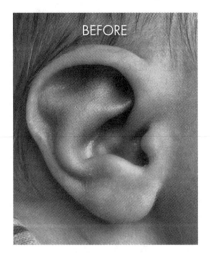 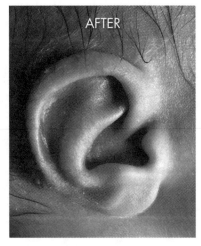

Photos courtesy of Dr. Yula Indeyeva.

Large, protruding ears that were not addressed with the splinting technique early enough in the child's life can be corrected at the age of six years. By that time, a child's ears have reached 90 percent of their adult size. Although this scenario is rare, if a child's nasal airway is obstructed as a result of a deviated nasal septum (the septum being the bone and cartilage in the midline of the inside of their nose), I recommend that the most minimal procedure necessary to correct the obstruction be performed. Otherwise, the facial skeleton may not develop normally.

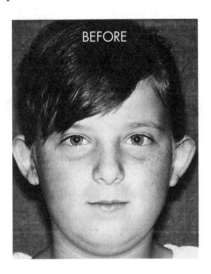
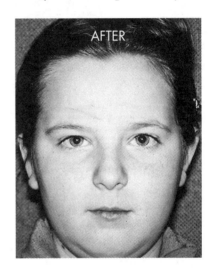

The Nose Factor

In most girls, a large or crooked nose can be corrected at the age of fifteen. Because boys usually mature later than girls, I recommend correcting boys' noses at sixteen years of age. These ages are not absolutes. I use them as general guidelines. There are ways to determine whether an adolescent has matured enough (both emotionally and physically) to undergo nasal plastic surgery. I should stress that emotional and psychological factors are as important as the physical ones and must be considered by all concerned, including the surgeon consulted.

With girls, I use two criteria. One is whether they have been having their periods on a regular basis for at least a year. With boys, I wait until they have needed to shave their facial hair for at least a year. With both genders, I like to wait until their shoe size is not changing every six months. The approach I take to this part of my practice follows the condition-specific approach that I take in all other aspects of it: I evaluate the conditions present and develop a treatment plan designed to specifically address them.

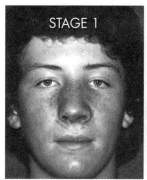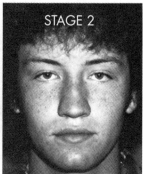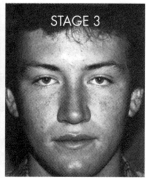

Repair of nasal fractures in a teenager.

The Chin Factor

Correcting a small chin by inserting a medical-grade implant underneath the skin and muscle of the front portion of a patient's mandible can provide balance in the facial features of both young women and young men. I describe this procedure in greater detail in chapter 13 of this book.

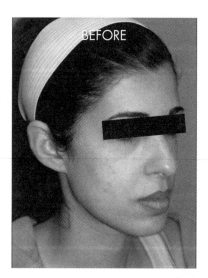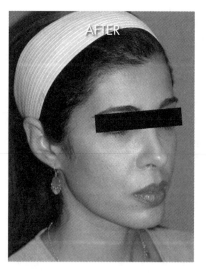

Chin and cheek augmentations.

A more invasive way to address unaesthetic chin conditions is to detach the lower portion of the mandible beneath the lower lip, slide it forward, and fix it with medial grade screws or plates. This operation is called "genioplasty" and is sometimes combined with correcting the bony unbalances of the midface. Craniofacial or orthognathic surgeons generally perform these procedures in conjunction with orthodontic therapy (braces and other devices applied to straighten the teeth).

To help determine whether a larger chin will enhance your self-esteem, a temporary measure can be tried. Some of the longer-lasting fillers can be injected beneath the muscle of your skin. While this course of action is not permanent and is not as dramatic as surgical chin augmentation, it is a consideration for the person not completely convinced that a larger chin is what they want.

Troubling Skin Conditions of Youth

Young men and young women alike are apt to develop acne during their maturing years. The emotional and psychological scars caused by the infected oil glands that cover their faces can be as troubling as the physical ones. Today, there are medications and treatments that can minimize the breakouts and any scarring that might result. When the side effects of Accutane can be tolerated, the drug can provide dramatic improvement in patients suffering from acne. Intense pulse light (IPL) treatments can also provide improvement. If scars should follow, I have found that a level 2 or 3 dermabrasion (not level 1 microdermabrasion) is the best method for improving such scars.

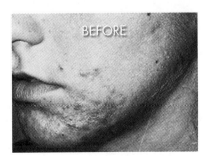 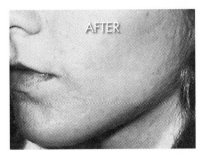

Level 3 dermabrasion to treat cystic acne.

Unsightly Scars

Improving scars caused by injuries falls under the category of reconstructive surgery and is a science unto itself. One of the paradoxes of wound healing is that incisions and cuts heal and mature more rapidly after the age of fifty than they do in children. The younger the child, the longer it takes for scars to flatten and for the pink discoloration that occurs with healing to dissipate.

As addressed previously, I usually tell my patients or their parents that in a two-year-old, an injury might take two to three years to pass through the phases of healing, whereas in a twenty year old, the same injury might heal in a year. In a seventy year old, the scar will be barely visible in six months. The best explanation I can give is that as we age, our skin becomes thinner, and thicker skin scars more than thinner skin. Another factor is that when scars are stressed, they tend to protect themselves by forming more scar. It seems that when we were created, a process was installed to keep wounds from opening during physical activity. Children, of course, are usually more active than septuagenarians.

If scars become thick, raised, and painful (a condition known as a keloid or hypertrophic scar), a series of cortisone injections can reverse the process and allow them to soften and flatten. In severe cases, low-dose, pinpoint radiation therapy may also be effective.

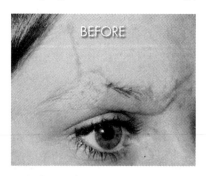 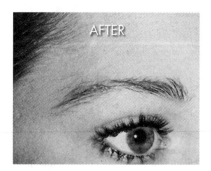

Augmenting Therapies for Young Lips

An ever-increasing number of young women under the age of twenty are consulting facial surgeons and dermatologists for neuromodulator treatments (Botox, Dysport, and Xeomin) as an attempt to prevent their faces from wrinkling in their older years. I am not an advocate of these treatments at such a young age, unless the injections are being used to treat migraine headaches. When used to address wrinkles, I recommend that my patients wait until they actually see early wrinkling before resorting to neuromodulator therapy. Vigilant sun protection is a safe way to prevent premature wrinkling and minimize the development of skin cancers in later years.

The truth is that those of us involved in the appearance-enhancing professions do not know the long-term effects of the frequent use of neuromodulators. I have been in practice long enough to see the detrimental effects of treatments that once were touted as "miracle treatments" for acne, such as the use of X-rays and ultraviolet light. It was not until decades had passed that the world discovered that almost every one of these patients developed invasive skin cancers in the areas treated. To add to the dilemma, when those cancers were removed, the incision sites were slow to heal and produced unsightly scars.

I'm not saying that the same phenomenon will occur with early and long-term use of neuromodulators; I am only saying that we do not yet know what the long-term effects are. So my advice is that you, as a young person or the guardian of a young person, err on the side of caution.

We are also seeing women age twenty or younger requesting that fillers be injected in their lips and other areas of the face. As long as the injections do not create grotesque-appearing lips, I can see no medical reason to deny them access to these treatments. As with any treatment, cost should be considered. If you add up the cost of having temporary injections placed in your lips, you will find that, from a financial point of view, within two to three years you will have spent more money than you would have had you undergone a permanent surgical correction.

For patients desiring fuller lips, I prefer to use small strips of their own collagen, taken from the crease behind their ears, to provide permanent bulk. In severe cases, a lip lift can be performed, with or without inserting a collagen graft.

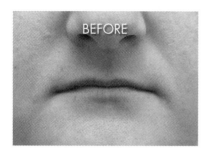 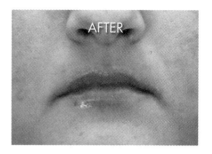

Augmentation and lip-line advancement surgery.

Fat injections are another possibility for women and men of any age. In my opinion, fat grafting is not yet as reliable as grafting carefully harvested strips of your own collagen.

Early Intervention in Skin Care

When it comes to professional skin care, I do not believe that you, your children, or your grandchildren can begin too early—within reason, of course. To help prevent and treat teenage acne, I recommend that you develop a good working relationship with a professional skin-care expert, just as you have likely done with a dentist. Periodic check-ups can often prevent big problems. For additional information about skin care, consult chapters 7 and 22–28.

Childhood and Adolescent Obesity

The number-one health risk affecting the younger generation of Americans is obesity. That's why I've devoted an entire chapter of this book to the subject. In chapter 8, I shared that I was fat as an adolescent. The scars embedded in my mind from comments made by my classmates and the shocking effect of seeing myself in that band photograph still linger. If you are a teenager, I urge you to give yourself the knowledge, inspiration, and encouragement needed to get your weight in line. If you are an adult who has sons, daughters, grandsons, or granddaughters who are overweight, give them the kind of loving advice they need to address their weight. Emphasize that, yes, it is hard. But managing your weight—at any age—is not an impossible task to master. Take it from me; the rewards will last a lifetime.

There are no age limits when it comes to initiating the processes that lead to becoming the best you can be. Starting young is just that: a start. It's a giant leap toward preventing conditions that can impair your ability to become the person of your dreams and therefore limit the opportunities that could be yours for the taking. The key to enjoying a lifetime of health, happiness, and prosperity is to keep giving yourself whatever gifts it takes for you to stay the course. And never refrain from seeking the assistance of professionals who possess the training, experience, and expertise necessary to assist you in expanding your horizons and becoming all that you were intended to be at the moment of your conception.

CHAPTER 34

Additional Self-Enhancement Measures

Now that we have explored the medicine and surgery of appearance enhancement, let's take a look at some of the other measures that can often provide what one of my facial plastic surgery mentors, Dr. Jack Anderson, liked to refer to as "the icing on the cake."

Wearing a Healthy Smile:
The Latest in Cosmetic and Implant Dentistry

Your smile speaks volumes about you. How you care for your teeth and gums is often a reflection of how you care for everything entrusted to you, including your mind, your body, your soul, and all those who depend upon you for their health and welfare.

Perhaps as much as in any field in the appearance and health industry, significant advancements have been made in the dental profession. No longer are dentists simply filling cavities and pulling teeth. Modern-day dental Rejuvenologists are able to help you maintain your dental health. The key is prevention of the conditions that cause your teeth to decay or become discolored.

Multiple factors influence the effectiveness of your personalized dental disease-prevention plan. As with many such plans, it begins with education. Knowledge about dental disease will help you understand how each preventive measure influences dental (and general) health. The more you know about the untoward consequences of neglect, the more motivated you become to implement preventive measures and find the dental professional best suited to meet your health and appearance expectations.

Regardless of your best efforts at home, it is important to establish a relationship with a dentist who can identify your individual needs, issue tailored instructions, monitor your efforts at home, and service both your needs and your desires. If your teeth and gums become diseased, the conditions can be treated and stabilized with professional assistance before they require more serious and expensive remedies.

Crooked teeth can be straightened. Darkened, stained teeth can be whitened. Broken or cracked teeth can be capped with natural-looking, long-lasting, laboratory-made prosthetic teeth attached to studs implanted in the bones from which teeth were removed. Finally, unattractive teeth can be shaped with orthodontic measures or camouflaged with aesthetically pleasing porcelain shields that look better than the teeth they shield.

The age of the removable denture is rapidly passing. Where teeth are missing, today's elite dental Rejuvenologists can implant anchoring devices deep in the gums and attach a permanent, natural-looking tooth or bridge (a prosthesis that contains multiple teeth) to the implants. Another bit of good news is that newer anesthetic techniques and technologically advanced equipment make the work performed by modern day dental Rejuvenologists virtually painless.

As a body owner, you owe it to yourself to maintain or create a healthy and aesthetically pleasing set of teeth—the underlying basis for a beautiful and confident smile. To learn more about cosmetic and restorative dentistry, consult a Rejuvenology-minded dentist.

The bottom line is this: do not underestimate how dentistry contributes to overall health and appearance. At some point in every human being's life, the condition of their dentition (mouth and gums) becomes an issue. As with other appearance-enhancing procedures addressed in this book, meticulous attention to and interpretation of each patient's expectations are critical to a happy outcome. When it comes to presenting your best self, careful communication about rejuvenating dental realities is as essential as the health component.

Currently, a plethora of flashy marketing campaigns promise one-stop solutions to complex dental problems. As has been often mentioned in other sections of this book—and exhibited through the history of the human race—"buyer beware" also applies to dentistry. A smile showing a poorly created set of teeth is as glaring as an overly operated nose, eyelids, or face. I remind you that several commercially focused organizations that spent millions of dollars advertising their franchised services have gone by the wayside, partially because franchise operations tend to hire inexperienced operators or operators who may have no other alternative.

Finally, a Rejuvenology dentist's aesthetic judgment is critical to the overall creation of beauty and harmony where neither may have previously existed. For example, an elongated face benefits from an appropriately wider dental complex in order to appear more pleasingly oval. Moreover, bold central incisors (eyeteeth) naturally draw attention to centrally located attractive features such as pretty, prominent lips. The myriad possibilities presented by the human face ensure the perpetual pursuit of educational excellence intrinsic to the dedicated cosmetic dentist.

Smarter Nutrition:
Its Positive Effects on Appearance and Health

Over the centuries, scientists have sought to identify the causative factors of diseases—the *reasons* they affect some of us and not others. Unlike infectious diseases that arise from causative microbial organisms (bacteria, viruses, fungi, etc.), other diseases are more complex. As a biochemical incubator, the body relies on building-block substances to generate energy. These substances are often referred to as the ingredients of life.

Foods consist of both macronutrients (larger components such as proteins, fats, and carbohydrates) as well as micronutrients (smaller components such as vitamins, minerals, antioxidants, enzymes, and probiotics).

These essential substances must counteract those that have a negative impact on the factors that control aging. Certain toxins are detrimental to the chemistry of life. Some of the most common include refined vegetable and seed oils, BPA (found in plastic food containers), trans fats (solid fats such as animal lard), red meat, coumarin (found in cinnamon), added sugar (especially from corn syrup), and mercury (found in fish).

In addition, two other chemically related reactions appear to speed the aging process: oxidation and inflammation. Both are influenced by the foods, supplements, and liquids we take into our bodies.

It can thus be concluded that the ability to control stress and inhibit inflammation is a gift a body owner can give to the cells all over their body. Another gift we can offer our bodies is to have annual complete metabolic profile examinations. Having a medical laboratory analyze a couple of vials of your blood can reveal vital information about your blood's levels of sugar, liver enzymes, immune proteins, lipids (cholesterol and triglycerides), prostate-specific antigen (PSA, related to prostate cancer), and C-reactive protein (a marker of blood vessel and cellular inflammation), as well as analysis of your white and red blood cell counts, thyroid function, and intracellular micronutrients. Changes in these tests over time signal abnormal metabolism long before the signs and symptoms of premature aging develop. By the time symptoms are present, treatment can be expensive and more difficult to correct.

Not until their bones become brittle do many people recognize the importance of calcium metabolism. A critical yet little-known fact is that 90 percent of people who suffer a broken hip after the age of seventy and are found to have osteoporosis (brittle bones) die within twelve months of the incident.

On the aesthetic side of the skeletal equation, posture is as important to appearance as any other factor. Furthermore, posture has everything to do with bone health, which is heavily dependent on balanced hormone levels as well as on metabolism of calcium and vitamin D. Nothing makes a person appear old and feeble more than bent-over posture coupled with a shuffling gait.

As potentially devastating as the condition may be, osteoporosis is largely preventable and treatable, assuming that the proper hormone replacement or medications are administered by a qualified medical professional. Nutritional testing for calcium and vitamin D levels coupled with bone-density screening every two years in people over forty are recommended to detect and treat bone loss.

Along with the bone-density exam, some doctors recommend taking posture photographs from both front and side views every two years. From such photographic documentation, you can tell if your posture has improved or if you are becoming stooped. Exercise, especially exercises aimed at strengthening your core (your abdomen and back) combined with effective stretching, such as yoga, Pilates, or the use of exercise balls, can go a long way in correcting the poor posture that often accompanies aging.

In terms of its impact on the signs of aging, gravity is relentless. Shrinking and bent posture are assured in the presence of weakened bones and muscles. Hormone-replacement therapy and calcium supplementation may be necessary to maintain good muscle strength in men and women.

Paracelsus (1493–1541) said, "From nature comes the disease, and from nature will come the cure." The Swiss physician did not mention that "nature" also includes your inherent ability to participate in obtaining and maintaining your health and appearance.

As previously mentioned, meals containing excess calories (more than those burned through physical activity) and diets high in simple sugars and saturated fat hasten disease and related aging processes. However, certain foods actually have healing and rejuvenating potentials. As a body owner, it is your responsibility to learn the difference and to follow guidelines that have been shown to foster well-being.

In specific ratios and amounts, amino acids (the building blocks of protein metabolism) may improve insulin and sugar metabolism, which has implications for diabetes and prediabetes. They may also lower blood pressure and cholesterol and improve fat cell cytokine balance. Proteins combined with food strategies that are specifically designed to control symptoms can often produce weight loss and improve well-being. The reason is that proteins take longer to be converted into the simple (natural) sugars that the cells of your body need in order to function properly. Thus, foods high in protein prevent the hunger and cravings that routinely follow the ingestion of simple carbohydrates (refined sugars). In addition, your body actually burns calories when it metabolizes protein or fat. It does not do so when you ingest refined sugars, which go directly into your bloodstream and cause a sudden outpouring of insulin in an attempt to neutralize the suddenly high levels of sugar.

Foods high in omega fatty acids, such as fish and nuts, reduce inflammation and oxidative stress. Vegetable oils (such as olive or canola oil) also reduce oxidative stress. These health-promoting oils (fats) may also be taken in high doses in pill or capsule form. Not all fats are bad for the body. Fats derived from animal food sources appear to be less favorable to human health and well-being. So if you are going to eat meat, trim the fat away, and try to stick to meats that do not have high concentrations of fat (which the meat industry refers to as being "marbled"). For example, a New York strip steak has less fat in the edible portion than does a rib-eye cut.

Fruits and vegetables are high in protective antioxidants. They also contain micronutrients that are necessary to the process of controlling inflammation. They also provide fiber for gut (stomach and intestinal) bacteria that produce protective anticancer and anti-inflammatory proteins.

Whole fruits and vegetables provide the complete package of fiber and micronutrients, whereas processed juices and extracts may not. Some fruit juices in particular may add to the negative impact of simple sugars on the body and promote inflammation.

As many myths surround food as facts about the realities. One of those facts is that segments of the self-help industry have learned to package the messaging about foods in ways that benefit their financial bottom lines more than the customers searching for answers.

You owe it to yourself to learn about foods, supplements, and metabolism. In addition to the information I provide in this book, you might want to consult a qualified nutrition counselor. The internet is a good place to gather questions for your counselor or health provider; however, it is not wise to make treatment decisions from internet information alone. A good starting point is the USDA site MyPyramid, located at FNS.USDA.gov/MyPyramid.

CHAPTER 35

Feeling as Well as You Look:

The Superior Doctor's Role

In the broadest sense, "doctor" means "teacher, or learned person."[11] This is reflected in the following ancient Chinese proverb, which has somehow lost its way in what is often referred to as "mainstream medicine":

> "The superior doctor prevents sickness.
> The mediocre doctor attends to impending sickness.
> The inferior doctor treats actual sickness."

Although it has long been accepted that prevention is better than cure, it seems that in the halls of government and in the boardrooms of Big Pharma and hospitals, prevention has taken a back seat to cure. "Learned" men and women have fallen prey to the wheels of the medical-industrial complex.

In my definition of superior doctors I include learned individuals and healers who are not physicians but who practice mind/spirit techniques as well as the intelligent use of vitamins, minerals, and herbs. Here it is important to establish an incontestable truth: vitamins, minerals, and herbs are not foods. Nor are they substitutes for food. Rather, they are micronutrients. In the right combinations and doses, they combine with the body's natural enzymes to assist in the metabolism of the foods—macronutrients—that are necessary for the body to assist itself in the integrative process known as healing.

In my professional opinion, nutritional supplements should not be used as a substitute for traditional medical and surgical care. However, they may serve a valuable adjunctive role in addition to traditional care

---

11. *Webster's New World College Dictionary*, 3rd ed. (1988), s.v. "doctor."

if and when deficiencies in either are identified. When cellular levels of a given vitamin, mineral, amino acid, or herb are optimal (better than normal), the cells of our bodies are better able to do what they were created to do: ward off disease. In cases where integrative care was also administered, marked enhancement of so-called traditional medical protocols may be observed.

The following testimonial makes the point for which I have been laying the necessary groundwork. It summarizes a real-life example in which mainstream medical professionals, adjunctive health profession-als, a committed patient, and his healer-trained wife worked both inside and outside government-mandated regulations in order to convert a traditionally fatal situation into a happy outcome. The story I share is that of Fiona and Jens Steffen. Fiona is a Registered Healer in the United Kingdom's National Federation of Spiritual Healers (the Healing Trust). About her husband's case, Fiona writes:

In June 2018, my seventy-eight-year old husband complained he felt he wasn't digesting his food properly and it felt heavy in his stomach. He was admitted to hospital with jaundice and a weight loss of six-teen pounds on July 14. So started a roller coaster of tests and scans.

A pancreatic mass was found at the head of his pancreas; his blood tests were grossly abnormal. His bile duct was blocked by the two-and-a-half-inch tumor. So, as a temporary solution, an (artifi-cial) drain was inserted, to allow the bile to flow.

Ten days later, he was discharged with the jaundice resolved; however, the results of a pancreatic cancer blood test remained well above the normal range. So, I took him home and immediately started him on two blended concoctions, consisting of twenty-one herbs, four times daily.

I also contacted a friend, a fellow Registered Healer, and asked her to send healing. Distant healing is a process in which a healer engages in an active participation with "the Source" (the entity most of us identify as God) and asks the Source to send healing energies to an absent person. Utilizing a variety of techniques that my healer friend and I were given, the two of us sent healing transmittals to Jens each day. As Jens's wife, I also resolved to make his last weeks or months the most joyous.

Despite the admonitions of well-meaning friends and relatives who suggested he become vegan or go on a raw food diet, my husband ate whatever he wanted. Food that had not been seen in our home often became regular staples: white bread, sugar—anything that was delicious and comforting.

By the last week of August, my husband was told by the specialists that he had no more than a year to live and that because the tumor was located so near the portal vein (the major vein that leads to from the liver to the heart), it was inoperable. We were told by mainstream specialists that Jens might have two years, but only if he underwent a course of chemotherapy to shrink the tumor. So, consulting an oncologist was his best chance to prolong his life.

Knowing what I know about healing and alternative therapies that have yet to be accepted as "evidence based" by the medical profession, Jens and I decided that with the clearly documented side effects of chemotherapy, Jens's quality of life would be diminished. Nevertheless, we agreed to meet with the oncologist.

Just a week before this meeting, my husband underwent a diagnostic test—a positron emission tomography (PET) scan. It is one of the best ways to identify cancerous tissue and determine if—and where—Jens's cancer might have spread.

By this time Jens, had lost thirty-eight pounds and was so weak he required a wheelchair to get him to the oncologist's appointment. From the waiting room, we were called in calmly and expected the worst. It took some time for the oncologist's words to register. He just kept repeating, 'This is very rare. The PET scan showed that the cancer was gone.'

Because of his age, state of health, and prognosis (by mainstream measures), the United Kingdom's National Health System (NHS) had written off my husband for any surgical treatment. So, even though the PET scan showed no cancer, we decided to go outside the NHS and opt for surgical confirmation. We approached one of the leading private pancreatic surgeons in the UK.

At the end of September—just one month later—we consulted with the pancreatic surgeon. Unlike when Jens required a wheelchair to visit the oncologist, after a further month of blended herbal drinks and healing thoughts sent his way, my husband, with renewed strength, color, and vigor, walked unattended into the surgeon's office.

Based upon the results of the previously performed PET scan, the surgeon agreed to perform a Whipple operation outside the National Health System. The Whipple operation is an extremely complex procedure during which part of the stomach, the gallbladder, part of the small intestine, part of the bile duct, and half of the pancreas is removed. Then the surgeon would rejoin what was left of the stomach to the small intestine.

This seven-hour operation took place in the middle of October. Instead of the usual seven to fourteen days, Jens spent only three days in intensive care and was then moved to the ward. By day five, he walked two hundred yards and climbed three flights of stairs. One week after the day of his surgery, he was discharged. Histological studies of the PET scan "hot spots" taken during surgery showed no cancer. We are told by doctors far and wide that such a case of "spontaneous remission" from pancreatic cancer is unheard of.

On follow-up visits to his surgeon, Jens has been told he has another twenty years to live. All the tumor was taken, with clear margins and all abnormal cells removed. We have been home for four weeks; each day he is stronger and eats whatever he likes. He has had no complications but will require three to four months to regain his full strength. It appears the specialists have not encountered a case like this before.

As a certified healer, I believe it is an example of the healing powers of thought, prayer, and mainstream and adjunctive medical procedures and potions, including:

- *My husband's extraordinary determination, mind-set, and dignity in accepting whatever came.*
- *Allowing a nonjudgmental, joyous time to occur.*
- *Providing anything he wanted, whether it was food or loving surroundings.*
- *Friends praying for him.*
- *Healing thoughts being sent by those of us who believe in their power.*
- *Healing herbs given daily.*
- *The body being allowed to relax with stress removed.*

The end result: an extraordinary miracle.

I would like to say my faith carried me, and on some days, it did. In my heart, I believed it would be all right; but at other times, I had accepted as reality that I would be spending Christmas alone.

Certainly, any human being's innate personal healing power is greatly underestimated. By stepping aside from the maelstrom of modern medicine and listening to the quiet inner voice, my husband and I reached a true healing experience.

Having said that, we are eternally grateful to the wonderful surgeon who used his expertise to perform a highly complex operation and follow-up care to fully resolve the problem and give Jens a full life span.

I believe the way forward is a collaboration of open minds between patients and the medical profession. We were fortunate to have found this in the end with an exceptional consultant surgeon— one willing to listen—when so-called "mainstream" medicine could not help or show an interest in adjunctive healing techniques and preparations used in a more holistic treatment plan.

Unless medical students are made aware of integrative (mind/body/spirit) medicine, and unless individuals of the human race are apprised of their own role in the quest for good health and well-being, how can this generation of healers be expected to know that other cost-effective, care-efficient ways to improve the quality and longevity of life exist?

Unfortunately, many modern day medical schools pay little attention to the patient's role in their health and well-being—and even less to the spiritual forces that are forever available. Unless medical schools take the lead by expanding their curricula to include what the "superior doctors" of China knew nearly four thousand years ago, how can physicians and physician extenders (nurse practitioners and physicians assistants) expect the public to become participating partners in the expanded health-care team of the future? Who will encourage people from all walks of life to embrace the healing powers in their minds, dormant but anxiously waiting to be roused? Who will make sure that integrative medicine (also known as holistic Rejuvenology) does not get lost again in the rush to replace hands-on caregiver/patient experiences with impersonal technology? Who—or what—will see that a body owner's health and well-being is a gift that humankind has not only the opportunity to give itself but the obligation? Who will impress upon tomorrow's physicians and allied health-care associates that when their future patients incorporate all the things that are required to look their best, those patients tend to find better health, even if finding better health was not the reason they chose to include appearance-enhancing procedures and products in their life plan?

I am a physician who has participated in medical sciences providing care from the first breath to the autopsy; who has worked within and outside third-party health care; and who believes that personal responsibility and unwavering faith are critical to maintaining the health of individuals and of a nation. Even so, try as I may, I am unable to see how government-managed health care as it is taking shape at the time of this writing will instill personal responsibility into the equation.

Healing-directed thought is not only a gift; in my mind, it is part of the definition of self-care—the kind of care readily available to every body owner at no additional cost. It is a large part of assisting every body owner as they move ever closer to becoming the person of their dreams.

CHAPTER 36

Your Body, in Shape, in All the Ways Possible

Many of the patients who ultimately made their way to my institute for appearance and health had embarked upon previous fitness programs in the same manner they began previous unsuccessful diets: by responding to an ad or commercial or by taking the advice of a friend, neighbor, or family member.

A case that comes to mind is that of a woman that you have already met, the one who was a hundred pounds overweight and who suffered from type 2 diabetes, high blood pressure, and hypercholesterolemia. Throughout most of her adult life, her weight had been a victim of the yo-yo phenomenon. She'd lose twenty pounds on some commercial diet plan, only to gain thirty pounds back. She'd join a fitness center with good intentions, only to lose interest in a few weeks. Although she searched, she never found the right combination of dieting and exercise, because she had failed to change the one thing that mattered: her *attitude* toward eating and exercise. It was the phenomenon of mind over matter that she had refused to embrace on an ongoing basis.

Following a surgical procedure to reduce the size of her stomach to approximately a third of its normal size, she lost her excess weight and saw her diabetes and high blood pressure disappear. Even so, she failed in the only measure that really matters to an obese individual. Although her stomach was unable to hold a full meal at any given time, she chose not to abandon her insatiable appetite for food and still ate all the things she craved, and more frequently.

This woman's experience is not uncommon. I know dozens of other friends and patients who have undergone stomaching reducing and in-testinal rerouting procedures only to regain most—if not all—the weight they originally lost.

It has been many years since I've seen my former employee, but I understand that she, too, has gained back all or most of the weight she lost. Hopefully, she will take the wise route going forward and choose to return to the person she was when she looked better, felt better, and was healthier, as is clearly obvious in the photographs below.

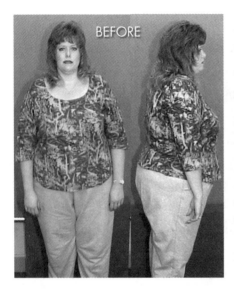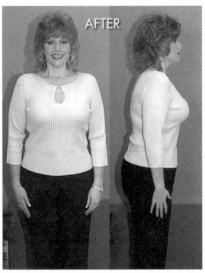

I pray that somehow this book, or at least its message, will find its way into her hands and mind and that she will assemble a team of professionals who will assist her in once again becoming the person she was in the photographs above—a person who exuded self-pride in all the ways it can be measured. I hope that she once again achieves that same look; that same expression of confidence; that enhanced state of health. I hope that she will do whatever it takes to maintain that state of being for the remainder of her life. For *her* sake, that is my wish.

In becoming the person of your dreams, your needs and tolerance may not be the same as mine or anyone else's. The prudent course of action is for you to consult a health professional and ascertain the condition of your heart and joints prior to embarking on a physical fitness program. Personal physicians, sports medicine professionals, internists, or cardiologists are best qualified to perform such evaluations. These professionals are usually associated with other therapists who may prove helpful in developing the ideal fitness prescription for every body owner.

To assist you in finding the right fitness expert for you, I offer the following recommendations.

It is an absolute fact that people view and judge you by your appearance, grooming, and posture. They also judge you by your balance, symmetry of shape, movement, and posture (BSMP). These physical attributes are also visible (or, as Dr. Marden puts it, "out-pictured") signs of health, and in many respects they are ours for the making. Face the facts: a healthy, vital appearance is more attractive than a stooped, aging, and needy one. As Aristotle wrote, "A pleasing appearance is more important than any letter of introduction." The celebrated philosopher and learned man was saying that the way you look when you walk through the door can open other doors of opportunity, including happiness, prosperity, and longevity.

The concept we glibly refer to as "balance" is complicated. Balance has to do with how the right side of the body moves with left; how the top moves with the bottom; how the front is proportional to the back; and whether one's posture gives off the impression of being strong, proud, and stable. Consciously or subconsciously, when one person's eyes scan another, whether or not they are aware of it, they are checking for the balance that another "learned man," Leonardo da Vinci, described balance and harmony in his Vitruvian Man. Keep in mind that the same balance and harmony criteria apply to women. Since balance indicates wholeness, stability, and vitality, it is an indicator of one's ability to function in whatever arena is called for. Clearly, balance (in all the ways it is measured) becomes more important as we age.

Symmetry—a concept similar to harmony—is a bit more complicated. Genetic factors play a role in each body owner's habitus, a term used to describe our proportionally measured physical shapes. Ideally, biceps should equal triceps. Hamstrings should equal quads. Buttocks should be proportional with abs. Shoulders and hips should fit in a triangle.

I once read, "If you want to discover a new idea, read an old book." To underscore this venerable truth, I remind you that Leonardo da Vinci's previously described depiction of the ideal proportions of the human body, the Vitruvian Man, was inspired by the work of first-century Italian Marcus Vitruvius Pollio.

I interpret Leonardo's and Vitruvius's messages to those they'd never know to mean that symmetry predicts balance because balance requires symmetry. Symmetry and balance predict and indicate movement ability. Pay attention to this phenomenon the next time you are sitting in an airport, train terminal, or shopping mall. Watch how people walk and move. You'll see just how observant Leonardo and Vitruvius were.

Movement and posture are closely related. When walking, it is important for a person who is in the fourth quarter of their life to exhibit a gentle side-to-side sway rather than a falling-forward cadence. Other tips for presenting a positive balance image include:

- Stand without rocking forward when rising from sitting.
- Accelerate smoothly into a walk or run.
- Turn and bend with control via core strength and balance.
- Strive to maintain stamina and endurance.
- Be ever aware of yourself.

Movement predicts function, and high-level function predicts social, economic, and spiritual aptitudes and abilities. Good posture—whether when sitting, standing, or walking—sends a message to the world that you are proud to be you and that you have given yourself the best chance to put your best self forward. The two unprompted postures demonstrated in the photographs of my former employee underscore this point. Note the sense of pride and balance this woman exhibits following the loss of more than one hundred pounds of excess weight. By losing this weight, she also rid herself of type 2 diabetes, high blood pressure, and high cholesterol.

A Personalized Fitness Plan

Being fit (in all the ways addressed in this book) is a gift that you can give to yourself. If you are an experienced exerciser, you may be able to assess your BSMP (balance, symmetry of shape, movement, and posture) on your own. If you are not qualified to do so, seeking counsel from a professional fitness or life coach is not only advisable but evidence that you are heeding the things you have learned in previous chapters. This is an indication that you are on your way to becoming the person of your dreams.

Good balance requires exceptional core strength in the muscles of both the abdomen and the lower back. For optimal results, however, it requires strengthening all muscles, top and bottom, front and back, right and left. Symmetry is similar: top and bottom, front and back, and right to left. Some women with extremely large and heavy breasts find themselves straining to stand erect for long periods of time. Many of these women choose to have breast reduction surgery and find that in addition to improving their appearance, the surgery also enhances their lives and sense of well-being.

Symmetry may also require losing excess fat through dieting and exercise or having some of it surgically removed with liposuction. Symmetry can also be enhanced by building muscle (body building) and balance-oriented exercises, such as yoga and Pilates.

Movement requires strength and balance: strong core muscles (abs) and strong limbs. Movement also requires endurance and stamina: aerobic capacity and muscle endurance.

As you are beginning to see, your optimal exercise program requires planning, strategy, and persistence. Here's how it works. With the end in sight, visualize what you want to achieve. Write it down—and be realistic. For example, any reasonable individual would rightly think that I am not in touch with reality if I were to include, on my own list of dreams, that I wanted to run a nine-second hundred-meter dash or a four minute mile, or clear a seventeen-foot pole vault bar, or win the Most Valuable Player Award in next year's Super Bowl, or hit the game-winning home run in next year's World Series, or make the winning free throw in the National Basketball Association's final game, or win the Masters golf tournament, or accomplish some other iconic feat.

So, notwithstanding the Broadway musical's message, my message to you is to appreciate the *Man of La Mancha*—Don Quixote's "impossible dream"—for the message it conveys but to focus on a realistic set of *possible* dreams in keeping with your own set of talents. In doing so, I recommend that you:

- Investigate the available possibilities.
- Focus on the ones that have a high probability of success.
- Plan the necessary techniques.
- Hire professional assistance, if needed.
- Get your mind in tip-top shape.
- Relentlessly, but wisely, implement your plan.
- Assess your progress on an ongoing basis.
- Make whatever adjustments your assessment determines are necessary.

The game plan summarized above is not new. In fact, it is extrapolated from the "winning theory" of the most-winning college football coach of his generation, Paul W. "Bear" Bryant. His methods proved to be more than theory, for my teammates and I were coached to apply them on and off the field of play. Because we faithfully bought into and followed our coach's plan, each of us was awarded a national championship ring at the conclusion of the 1964 college football season.

Students and fans of college football can see the same principles that won for Coach Bryant's teams at work on autumn Saturdays, when Coach Nick Saban's Crimson Tide take the field.

If you are just embarking on a personal enhancement program and your muscles and joints are not accustomed to the kind of use and stress you will require of them, you could injure yourself. So, start slowly and work your way up gradually. Every championship bodybuilder, gymnast, or rodeo champion did so. Muscle strength and balance are neither created nor recaptured overnight. Like other factors that recapture youth and appearance, physical fitness is a process.

For the noncompetitive athlete or dancer, a reasonable exercise program does not necessarily require a lot of time. You'd be surprised how a results-focused routine that challenges all muscle groups performed for ten to twelve minutes daily will yield results within two to three weeks.

Keeping Score

As with any goal-oriented task, measuring the accumulating results of a fitness program reinforces the mission—one based upon a healthy balance between efforts exerted versus results achieved. Just as you look in the mirror to see improvement after cosmetic surgery or injectable fillers, so should you look in the mirror, at photographs, or at measuring devices to realize the benefits of fitness-based body-shaping and balance efforts.

Balance is the easiest of all impressionable elements to enhance and measure. The simplest method is to stand on one foot a couple of times per day. Time yourself. When the other foot touches the floor, record the amount of time elapsed. Measure three times, and take the average. Measure this average monthly when you start your exercise program. As core balancing muscles are stimulated, so shall they respond.

Symmetry is best monitored by a series of photographs. Stand in front of something that allows for measurement: a doorframe, bricks along the wall of the house—something with symmetry against which you can compare future photographs. Snap frontal and side-view photographs to evaluate your posture. Take new photographs every six months, and compare the results of your efforts. As with other conditions addressed in this book, the fact that you are becoming more aware of your posture will cause you to enhance it.

Movement is measured by stride and distance. Look at your footprints. How straight is your stride? What is your maximum stride length at maximal walking speed? How far can you walk or run without stopping to rest?

When engaging in fitness and balance activities, you should pay attention to your body. This is an admonition that I share with each of my patients before and after appearance-enhancing surgery. I say it in a slightly different way: "Listen to your body. It will tell you if you are doing something that you are not quite ready to do."

Through feedback mechanisms built in at the time of conception, our bodies will warn us when they are being stressed beyond current limits. These are times when the adage "no pain, no gain" can result in disastrous consequences. Pain is one of the ways a body tells its owner that it is testing the limits. Young bodies are better equipped to handle the "no pain, no gain" principle. Body owners beyond the age of thirty should listen closely to their bodies. If you are one of them and experience sudden pain while engaging in physical activities, immediately *stop* whatever you are doing and rest. There are times when "no pain, no gain" may produce more harm than good. The educated and experienced body owner knows that continuing on in the face of pain may produce further injury.

You should measure the point in your fitness regimen where you experienced pain. Pay close attention to how long or how far you have exercised. More importantly, you should seek medical attention if you experience pain in your chest, shoulder, arm, or jaw, even if the pain goes away when you stop doing what you were doing.

Without attempting to come across as an alarmist, I remind you that I identify as a pragmatist. If you have experienced any of these symptoms while engaging in physical or stressful activities, a cardiologist may recommend a stress test, during which you can be monitored by an EKG machine to see whether your heart is healthy enough to continue with the program you have been previously prescribed. While stress tests can indicate how far you can go before subjecting your heart to a heart attack, a calcium score performed on your heart with a simple CT scan can more accurately determine if, where, and to what degree your coronary arteries are obstructed.

The next step in documenting the results of a CT-assisted calcium score is a noninvasive angiogram, during which a dye is injected into one of your arm veins. As the dye passes through you coronary arteries, the scanner records the location and degrees of blockages, if any exist.

Some cardiologists prefer to insert a small catheter into one of the larger veins in your groin, thread the catheter into the coronary arteries, and inject the dye. If obstructions to your coronary arteries are identified, many cardiologists will immediately insert an expanding stint to open the arteries in places where narrowing is discovered.

I hope that my reasoning for including these revelations in this book is becoming what the Founding Fathers of America described as "self-evident." I want you to be better informed about conditions and measures related to your overall well-being.

When it comes to symmetry, balance, exertion, and keeping score, simple measures work, but as with everything you (as a body owner) are expected to consider, unless you write your goals down and refer to them often, you are apt to see the realization of them disappear before your eyes—as do many of "the best laid plans of mice and men." This phrase, used by John Steinbeck in the title of his 1937 novel *Of Mice and Men*, derives from Scottish poet Robert Burns's "To a Mouse." Burns was inspired by the sight of the nest of a family of mice disappearing before his eyes while tilling a field of wheat. It is a message for the ages, one also reflected in the Yiddish phrase "Mann Tracht, Un Gott Lacht"—"man plans, and God laughs." The literal meaning is this: despite our most careful planning, the road of life is unpredictable.

So how do the admonitions of ancient Judaism, a Scottish poet, and a twentieth-century American novelist apply to a book dedicated to the principle that you have within yourself the ability to become the person of your dreams? If you are still reading, you know the answer. While you can plan, include the wisdom of the ages, exert the necessary energies, and ask for guidance from the Source, life may still serve up lemons from time to time. The best you can do is to squeeze them for all they are worth and make lemonade. Along the way, you are also expected to use the gift of reason to know when to stop squeezing.

CHAPTER 37

Your Enhancement Prescription

Although each of our genes can ostensibly be traced back to a single Source and a pair of divinely engineered human beings, every one of us is slightly different from the next. Because of many of the factors I have addressed in this book, the same body is different from year to year, constantly changing with age. With that fact in mind, every part of our life-enhancement programs should be customized to our condition-specific body skills and objectives. Each aspect of our plan should be reassessed on a periodic basis and when unanticipated circumstances suddenly present themselves.

Before embarking on a mind/body/spirit enhancement program, you should remember that every cell in your body is in a constant stage of replicating itself and then dying off to make room for its clone. As you factor this fact into your life plan, ask yourself the following questions:

- What is this constantly renewing body that I am going to give myself going to do for me?
- Will it give me more self-confidence?
- Will it allow me to interact more with those I love?
- Will it allow me to advance in my profession or job?
- Will it help me attract a companion or mate?
- Am I committed to maintaining the improvements I achieve?

I strongly recommend that you write down your answers. It will take only a few minutes. Think how important those minutes will be compared to the hours, days, weeks, and months of time and energy you commit to becoming the person of your dreams, cell by cell, at every age.

The Fitness Professional's Role

As with other components of your life plan, once your physical fitness goals are specifically outlined, review them with a professional exercise instructor. Schedule an hour to review your objectives, health limitations, exercise knowledge, timelines, and cost—*and be painfully honest*. Have your prospective instructor weigh in on how realistic the goals you have set for yourself are, and make sure they fit with the other aspects of your lifelong enhancement plan. The time and money spent in this session could be the best expenditure you ever make.

I recommend that you refrain from being like most people, who show up at the gym and just start exercising without a condition-specific mission in mind. Seek professional guidance and coaching until you are able to plan and implement your own program. At least at the beginning, it is wise to make sure you are not alone when you engage in strenuous exercise. If you are alone, keep your cell phone handy. Accidents and events happen, and if someone is present, within shouting distance, or accessible via phone, it could save your life, as it did for a friend of mine.

A colleague of mine in facial plastic surgery recently collapsed on the way to his car after playing tennis with a fellow physician. It was fortuitous that he had chosen a fellow physician as his playing partner. His colleague was able to perform CPR until the 911 paramedics arrived on the scene. As they are trained to do, the paramedics continued the life support exercises until the doctor—who had suddenly become a patient in distress—arrived at the emergency department of the nearest hospital. He was immediately taken to the cath lab, where stints were placed in his coronary arteries. A few days later, the doctor, who had suffered a cardiac arrest, walked out of the hospital, and he is back doing what he does best—helping his patients enhance their appearance and well-being.

Was it coincidence that my friend and fellow facial plastic surgeon selected another physician for his tennis partner, or did he give himself the gift of life by wisely considering the potential consequences of strenuous exercise after the age of forty and planning accordingly? Since retired major general David Bockel convinced me that "there are no coincidences," I contend that my medical colleague's life was saved because of decisions he made prior to the cardiac event.

Wisely selecting the people with whom you choose to associate as you engage in the game of life could be yet another hedge against genetically driven premature aging. Intelligently exercising your various body systems on an ongoing basis is another of those gifts that you can give yourself—another way to exercise self-care and delay the predisposition to genetically linked diseases.

Because I have long known the mind-set of my colleague who suffered a cardiac arrest in the parking lot of a tennis court, I am convinced that the reason he was able to overcome an event that might have had a different outcome for the less-committed segment of our society was because he was a frequent participant in physical activity, had endured many of the challenges facing our specialty, and had a fighter's mentality.

In any respect, I am proud that my friend survived this life test and that I can share a happy outcome with you. I urge you to keep his story in mind as you embark on strenuous physical activity.

The Aerobic Factor

On the mental side of the comprehensive life-enhancement equation, prudently practiced physical activity has also been shown to reduce the stress that comes with competing in today's society. Physical activities tend to lower blood pressure, blood sugar, cholesterol, and triglycerides, the combination of which can lead to early debilitation and demise.

Burning hollow calories through physical exercise can also help you maintain a healthy weight. Yet not all physical activity is the same. Equal activities may not produce equal results. In addition to following the recommendations I have shared in this book, you may need the input of an exercise professional who is willing to work with your primary care physician to develop a condition-specific fitness program designed specifically with your well-being in mind.

Some experts believe that to obtain the cardiovascular benefits of exercise, the activity must be of an aerobic nature, meaning that your pulse rate must be raised to almost two times your resting rate and maintained at that pace for at least twenty minutes. Recent studies are recommending even longer sessions. That the debate is ongoing says to me that the final answer is not yet in. So, how long—and how often—you need to exercise is an ongoing dilemma. The bottom line is that *some* physical activity, carried out on a daily basis, is better than *no* physical activity, even if it means taking the stairs rather than the elevator, parking a bit farther away from the entrance of your destination, getting up out of your chair at least once every hour and exercising the muscles of your legs, or engaging in isometric exercises while delayed in traffic on your way to and from work.

As is the case with all things that affect our appearance, health, and well-being, moderation is the key. Too much of anything can be as detrimental as too little. An experienced and knowledgeable team of professionals can tailor a physical activity program that is right for you and your mission of becoming the person of your dreams. You might also want to resist purchasing exercise equipment prior to checking with your doctor and a personal trainer. Without knowing the appropriate exercise routine and weight limits for your body, you could injure yourself.

For decades, my medical colleagues believed that three twenty-minute sessions of aerobic exercise per week were adequate to keep your heart and blood vessels healthy. That's a total of one hour. More recently, some specialists have been recommending sessions lasting twice that long. The conflicting opinions touted by different respected medical sources makes it difficult for both you (as a consumer of health-related services) and me (as a physician) to know what to do. For example, long distance runners who run for hours per week sometimes die of heart attacks before the age of fifty. The case of Darryl Kile, a Major League Baseball player, also comes to mind. At the age of thirty-three, Kile died of a heart attack. It is important to add that he was a pitcher.

Anyone who has played baseball in high school (as I did) and beyond will tell you that baseball coaches require that pitchers and catchers be more physically fit than members of the team who play other positions. The reason is that on every pitch, pitchers and catchers not only are exerting energy but are placed in ongoing situations of mental stress.

When I played football for the University of Alabama, one of my teammates once grabbed his chest in the heat of a mentally and physically challenging practice and said aloud, "I think I'm having a heart attack."

One of the trainers casually walked over to the player and asked a few questions, then said, "You're all right." So my former teammate tried to continue, but he was unable to do so. Instead, he walked off the field, changed into his street clothes, and was never again seen on the practice field.

A few years later, I was told that he was drafted into one of the branches of the armed forces and, during his preadmission physical examination, was told that his EKG showed that he had indeed had a heart attack at some point in his young life. At the time, this man was only nineteen years old. Whether my former teammate's heart attack occurred that day in practice, we may never know; however, every year we read about high school and college athletes who die on practice fields.

So while exercise is an important factor, physical activity alone is not the answer to health, happiness, prosperity, and longevity. The stress factor cannot be overlooked. Even taking into consideration Darryl Kyle's incident, the collective benefits that arise from smartly executed and diligently practiced exercise and stress-relief programs appear to be well worth the efforts invested.

Examples of aerobic exercises include vigorous walking, jogging, swimming, and biking. Unless you have consulted your physician and a personal trainer, you should adopt a policy of "crawl, walk, and then run." Gradually work your way into an exercise routine, and—at least in the beginning—let the first sign of fatigue be your stopping point. Gradually work your way into a "no pain, no gain" routine.

Because it is not always necessary to have exercise equipment readily available, there is little reason to not engage in *some* aerobic exercise several times per week, even if it is just routinely taking the stairs on your way to and from work or walking up and down stairs during your coffee or lunch break.

Nonaerobic Exercise

Physical activities that cause you to produce bursts of energy in relatively short periods of time are known as nonaerobic exercises. Examples of nonaerobic exercises include lifting heavy weights, push-ups, sit-ups, sprinting, driving a defensive line off the line of scrimmage, power running or walking, and other creative bursts of energy that burn calories and stress your muscles. Nonaerobic exercises are designed to build and strengthen muscles, but they may not have the positive effect on your heart and cardiovascular system that, at this time in the history of the human race, aerobic exercises are believed to have. It stands to reason that sudden and severe bursts of energy raise your blood pressure and pulse rate to levels that could actually be detrimental to your heart, particularly if you are over the age of forty.

Contrary to what television and print advertisements might tell you, you don't need costly exercise equipment to strengthen and condition your heart and other muscles. Sit-ups, push-ups, knee bends, and isometric exercises can be performed anywhere you find yourself in the world at any time. You can even perform isometric exercises sitting in your car at stoplights or in traffic, in an airplane, on a train, at work while sitting at your desk, or while watching television.

I once had a former competitive body builder work for me. During one of our conversations, he shared how, when he was away from his gym, he relied upon isometric resistance exercises by creatively tugging on a towel from the bathroom of his hotel room to bulk up his muscles prior to competitive events.

If you're old enough, you might remember the Charles Atlas advertisements from the mid-1950s. His secret to changing his body from that of a skinny teenager who was bullied on the beach to a superman-like physique was based upon resistance exercises—engaging the muscles of contraction to strengthen the opposing muscles of resistance for eight to ten seconds.

Here's another case in point. When I played center on the University of Alabama's 1964 national championship team, my teammates and I were subjected to the Charles Atlas isometric system of strength building. The team's chief trainer convinced Coach Bryant that weight lifting produced bulk and that quickness—as opposed to body mass—was the way to neutralize opponents whose fitness programs were based upon nonaerobic weightlifting programs.

Whether the trainer's assessment was correct can be measured by the fact that during the time I played there, the University of Alabama's football teams won two national championships—more often than not against teams that were bigger than were we. In the ensuing three years, the university's teams went undefeated and won another national championship. At least for us, isometric exercises worked wonders.

Once again, the key to any health-oriented activity is knowing:

- What to do.
- How to do it.
- How often to do it.
- Why you are doing it.
- To what limits you should stress yourself.

That's why professional counseling and personalized instruction are crucial to obtaining desirable outcomes. One-on-one personalized assessment of your objectives and limitations accompanied with condition-specific training leads to better results and provides ongoing motivation and instruction.

From my personal experiences as an athlete and as a physician, I offer the following recommendation. Your ideal and personalized life-enhancement program should include a healthy balance of the various programs that I have shared with you throughout this book.

The Advantages of a Prescriptive Lifestyle

As with other factors in creating a beautifully balanced life, your prescriptive lifestyle program should not be looked upon as a one-size-fits-all regimen. The amount, nature, and intensity of the activities, products, and procedures recommended to you should be based on an objective mutually agreed upon by you, your life coach, your doctor, and other professionals whose opinions you respect.

Make sure you tell each member of your life-enhancement team whether you have any underlying health conditions that might be negatively affected by the products and programs to which you may be subjected on your way to becoming the person of your dreams.

Measuring and monitoring your progress is the way to keep score. Without accurate documentation, it is impossible to measure the success—or lack thereof—that you garner from the time and effort invested in a personalized life-enhancement program.

In a previous chapter, I explained how a successful weight-management program requires a lifelong commitment. Here, it is important to note that as your physical condition changes (through the aging process or unexpected events), so must every component of your life plan. This is another reason why a long-term professional relationship with a team of experts is crucial to maintaining the results obtained.

For example, if you suffer from chronic back or joint problems, you will require a different physical fitness program than someone not challenged by those conditions. Perhaps swimming or water aerobics should be in your plan. If you are hampered by documented coronary and heart disease, you might need to begin with a less strenuous series of activities and gradually work your way up to a more aggressive exercise program.

There are many reasons why any one-size-fits-all plan may not fit your individual needs and objectives. In like manner, the axiom "self-treatment is often poorly advised treatment" applies to appearance-enhancing procedures and products, exercise, vitamin and dietary therapy, and a plethora of other factors that play into becoming the person of your dreams. Self-care is another matter. It involves incorporating all the things you learn from the professionals you consult into an ever-evolving life plan.

For your own good, you should avoid adopting someone else's life-enhancement regimen as your own, especially if it involves policies and procedures that make you uncomfortable. First, be evaluated by the team of professionals addressed in previous sections of this chapter.

Reaching Your Potential: The Optimal Level for You

Once your own personalized life-enhancement prescription has been determined—and as your grit, your endurance, and your capacity to achieve more than you might previously have imagined increases—it will be time to reassess where you are in the game of life. Should you continue to press your luck? Should you take stock and say to yourself, "This is good. I'm OK where I am, doing what I am doing, right here." Or should you set new goals and continue to reach higher than you ever dreamed? I cannot answer these questions for you. You must answer them yourself. You have that gift. It was given to you at the time of your conception by the Source of all that is good and great. Our responsibility is to clearly identify the talents we have been given and to develop them to the best of our abilities without doing harm to ourselves or others. That is all we can do. I believe it is all we should aspire to do. And as we do what we can do, we must always listen to that little voice in the back of our mind saying, "Everything in moderation." I believe this is the voice of our spirit—the part of us that connects us with the Source of our being.

As you go forward in a world teeming with misinformation, keep the warning that I have stressed in this chapter and throughout this book at the forefront of your mind. In any process designed to enhance your appearance or health, it is possible to go overboard and, in one beat of your heart—perhaps its last beat—to lose to the ages the person that you have become.

CHAPTER 38

The Right and Wrong Reasons to Consult

Appearance-Enhancing Professionals

As I walked into my consultation room and greeted the young woman sitting in the chair across from my desk, I thought to myself, *Why is she here to see me?*

As is customary in my practice, I had already reviewed the pictures taken of the prospective patient by my photographer a short while earlier. Both in her photographs and in person, she was an attractive young woman. *Perhaps*, I thought, *she sees herself as a person in need of enhancement surgery. Perhaps she has body dysmorphic disorder.*

Taking a seat in the chair on my side of the desk, I began our conversation with, "Can you tell me why you are here?"

I'll summarize the rest of the conversation. She requested a small amount of improvement to her lips, nose, and cheeks. As I agreed that those parts of her face were slightly out of balance with her other features and recognized no obvious signs or symptoms of body dysmorphic disorder (BDD), I agreed to perform procedures to give her the minimal improvement I felt was indicated. Afterward, all her features were in compliance with Leonardo da Vinci's proportions of the ideal human face. I thought she would be elated with the outcome of the procedures I had performed. I know I was.

However, a few months later, the patient returned to my clinic and requested additional changes to her face and nose. During her visit, I demonstrated in a three-way mirror how her facial features were absolutely in balance. The harmony I thought she'd sought had been achieved. Nonetheless, my professional opinion fell on deaf ears. Her mind was already made up. She refused to see the true beauty the mirror reflected.

Because my patient could not see things as they were in the mirror, I showed her the improvement obtained through the procedures I had performed. I demonstrated how the minimal changes I had made to her face reflected a beautiful example of Leonardo da Vinci's criteria for ideal facial harmony. However, nothing I said or demonstrated mattered. In her mind's eye, she saw only an ugly face, and she pleaded with me to perform more surgery. She wanted her cheeks and lips made larger and her nose made smaller. She was willing to "pay whatever" I charged if I'd carry out her wishes. What she could not grasp was that it was never about the money; it was about doing—or *not* doing—the right thing. No matter how professionally and caringly I attempted to convince my patient of this, she left my office dissatisfied.

A year or so later, she returned. During the interim, she had found a surgeon who'd agreed to perform the additional surgeries she'd requested. Now her features no longer resembled the beautiful face I had seen during her previous visits to my clinic. She was rightly distraught and pleaded that I help her.

After she agreed to seek psychological counseling and convinced me that she would be satisfied if I removed the cheek implants inserted by the other surgeon and returned her lips to a more pleasing size, I agreed to correct the ill-advised and overdone surgery that had been performed by a colleague in another state.

Within a few weeks, the patient began emailing photographs to me and asking me to reinsert the cheek implants I'd agreed to remove and once again enlarge a lip that was, thanks to my corrections, in harmony with her facial features for the first time in a long time. Hers was a classic case of body dysmorphia—"a mental disorder in which [the afflicted individual] can't stop thinking about one or more perceived defects or flaws in [their] appearance—a flaw that, to others, is either minor or not observable. But [body dysmorphic individuals] may feel so ashamed and anxious that they may avoid many social situations."[12]

---

12. "Body Dysmorphic Disorder," Mayo Clinic, Mayo Foundation for Medical Education and Research, accessed September 30, 2019, https://www.mayoclinic.org/diseases-conditions/body-dysmorphic-disorder/symptoms-causes/syc-20353938.

In retrospect, I wish I had been more perceptive when this patient first asked me to alter her features. If I had suspected BDD, I would have refused to perform *any* appearance-altering surgery on her. The truth is that even with decades of experience in cosmetic medicine and surgery, I was fooled. I missed the diagnosis.

This patient's story underscores why, throughout this book, I focus on your mind, body, and spirit—for unless you know yourself inside and out, you may never be able to balance all three of the components of life that make you who you are. You may never be content with who you are and are capable of becoming.

I wish to emphasize several points about BDD. If you are a prospective patient or an appearance-enhancement professional, you should become familiar with the signs and symptoms of body dysmorphic disorder.

In previous chapters, I shared ways to enhance your appearance to improve your chances of prospering in a competitive world. I stressed that the key to enhancing your appeal index is moderation; extremes of too little or too much tend to detract from your appearance and your health. A person who suffers from BDD may seek appearance-changing procedures for the wrong reasons or at the wrong time in their life. These patients tend not to be aware of the fact that they suffer from BDD and continue to pursue appearance-altering procedures until they no longer resemble the person that they were when they embarked upon the process of changing the way they look. A person who suffers from BDD does not have a clear image of the person they would be happy as. They never seem to be comfortable in their own skin. Their idea of perfection continues to change as their appearance changes. There is no end, at least not until the end is one defined by tragedy. In my professional opinion, the late Michael Jackson was a classic example of BDD.

As an appearance-enhancing surgeon, I thought Michael looked great following his first two operations. As he continued to have more, however, he became a creation. He did not appear to be black or white, male or female. With each subsequent procedure, he developed the dreaded sequelae of overdone plastic surgery. Toward the end of his life, he turned from surgery to drugs. One drug in particular cost him his life.

As you review the signs and symptoms of BDD provided in the following paragraphs, you, too, will wonder whether Michael's reliance on drugs was his way of dealing with his condition. Sad as it was, his quest to become someone other than who he was turned out to be self-destructive.

In my own practice, I have consulted with patients who suffered from varying degrees of BDD. They tend to be great actors and are skilled at deceiving physicians. If I recognize the disorder (and in the vast majority of cases, I can), I recommend *against* surgery, at least until the patient provides a written release from their psychologist or psychiatrist indicating that they are acceptable candidates for appearance-altering surgery. Some of these patients actually do exhibit physical imbalances in their facial or body features that detract from their appearance. Once those conditions are brought into balance—and with psychological counseling—these patients are able to function normally in society. Other BDD patients continue to search until they find a surgeon or surgeons who agree to perform whatever procedures they request, without being cleared by their therapist.

To assist you in the assessment process, review this list of questions that you need to ask yourself and answer honestly and forthrightly.

- Are you extremely preoccupied with a perceived flaw in your appearance that others can't see or believe to be minor?
- Do you have a strong belief that you have a defect in your appearance that makes you ugly or deformed?
- Do you believe that others take special notice of your appearance in a negative way or that they mock you?
- Do you engage in behaviors aimed at fixing or hiding the perceived flaw that are difficult to resist or control, such as frequently checking the mirror, grooming, or skin picking?
- Do you attempt to hide perceived flaws with styling, makeup, or clothes?
- Do you constantly compare your appearance to that of others?

- Do you frequently seek reassurance about your appearance from others?
- Do you have perfectionistic tendencies?
- Do you seek frequent cosmetic procedures yet receive little satisfaction?
- Do you tend to avoid social situations?
- Are you so preoccupied with your appearance that it causes major distress or problems in your social life, at work, at school, or in other areas?
- Do you obsess over one or more parts of your body?
- Do you refuse to recognize that the feature that you focus on may change over time?
- Are you aware of the most common features over which people tend to obsess?
  - The face, including the nose, complexion, wrinkles, acne, and other blemishes.
  - Hair, including the appearance, thinning, and baldness.
  - Appearance of the skin and veins.
  - Breast size.
  - Muscle size and tone.
  - Genitalia.

Just because you identify with a few of the symptoms on this list does not mean that you suffer from BDD. Chances are that anyone reading this can identify with some of them. Once again, it is when things are taken to the extreme that they become pathological (detrimental to your health and well-being).

Perhaps body dysmorphia should be called pathological vanity, as it can impact sufferers with varying degrees of severity. Keep in mind that I consider vanity to mean that a person is so concerned about their appearance that it interferes with their ability to function normally in society. As you contemplate the list of symptoms again, ask yourself whether your beliefs about your perceived flaws are valid. You might conclude that the flaws you see are real but that you can live with them. Or, knowing that perfection is extremely rare, you might conclude that if you did choose to undergo surgery designed to address real imperfections, you could live with a result that ends up being less than perfect. The conclusions you reach matter, for they will indicate both to yourself and to the professionals you consult whether you have BDD and, if so, how severe it is.

The principle of early prevention applies to all manner of unhealthy conditions. The first line of defense is awareness. The second line is early detection. The third—and least effective—is treatment of the disorder *after* it has adversely affected your health and well-being. This is not a new concept. As previously mentioned, it was expressed in an ancient Chinese proverb nearly four thousand years ago. It just needs to be brought from the annals of history into the present. It needs to be taught throughout every nation's educational system, beginning in kindergarten. Every child should understand that the new way forward should be to take responsibility for your health, as well-being is a gift you give yourself. Imagine a world in which self-care becomes the new standard of care and prevention of sickness is the first line of defense. Reality will follow closely behind.

With that standard in mind, it is important to know that BDD typically starts in the early teenage years and affects both males and females. Muscle dysmorphia, an obsession with the idea that one's build is too small or not muscular enough, occurs almost exclusively in males.

Certain factors seem to increase the risk of developing or triggering BDD, including:

- Having blood relatives who have body dysmorphic disorder or obsessive-compulsive disorder.
- Negative life experiences, such as childhood teasing and trauma.
- Certain personality traits, such as perfectionism.
- Societal pressure or expectations of beauty.
- Having another psychiatric disorder, such as anxiety or depression.

As with many disorders, BDD often has short- and long-term complications, which can include:

- Major depression or other mood disorders.
- Suicidal thoughts or behavior.
- Anxiety disorders.
- Health problems from behaviors like skin picking.
- Obsessive-compulsive disorder.
- Eating disorders.
- Substance abuse.

A recent scientific study indicated that approximately 2–2.5 percent of Americans suffer with some degree of BDD.[13] On the surface, that might appear to be a small number, but the fact that it represents two Americans in every one hundred should serve as a wake-up call for appearance-altering providers and our prospective patients.

There's currently no known way to prevent body dysmorphic disorder. However, because BDD often starts in the early teenage years, prompt identification and treatment of the disorder may be of some benefit. Long-term maintenance treatment by trained therapists may also help prevent a relapse of the condition.

If you are considering any changes to your appearance or body, you should study the list of BDD signs and symptoms provided above. If you think that you or someone you care about might be in need of counseling, my advice is to aggressively pursue the matter *prior* to undergoing appearance-altering surgery. I have never believed that asking for help is a sign of weakness. On the contrary, it is a sign of strength and a clear indication that you truly are on your way to becoming the person of your dreams.

I am happy to report that the vast majority of people who seek appearance-enhancing procedures do not suffer from BDD or pathological vanity. Most are well-balanced individuals who seek my advice and present with realistic expectations. And, as you've learned from the stories

13. L. M. Koran, E. Abujaoude, M. D. Large, R. T. Serpe, "The Prevalence of Body Dysmorphic Disorder in the United States Adult Population," *CNS Spectrums* 13, no. 4 (April 2008): 316–22, https://doi.org/10.1017/s1092852900016436.

shared throughout this book, enhancing these patients' appearance also greatly enriched their lives and the lives of others.

The reason I chose to include body dysmorphic disorder at this point in this book is to emphasize the central message that balance, harmony, and symmetry are the keys to a life lived well and that anything taken to the extreme can be detrimental to becoming the person of your dreams.

CHAPTER 39

Gifts for the Taking

At the beginning of this book, I promised that if you kept an open mind and stayed with me to the very end, you would learn how to give yourself the ability to take charge of your life. I promised that if you followed the comprehensive life plan I advised, you would see the doors of opportunity swing open for you more widely than you might have imagined. I did not promise that enhancing your appearance, improving your health, and succeeding in a competitive world would be easy. On the contrary, I emphasized that *if* you adopted and diligently followed my recommendations, you would be on your way to becoming the you of your dreams—and then some.

- You would come to see yourself and the world around you through enlightened eyes.
- You would come to recognize and accept the things about yourself that you should not attempt to change, find the courage to make the changes that would enhance your appearance, health, and self-image, and come to know the difference.
- You would be better prepared to assemble a team of professionals to help you attain the kind of results and care that you expect.
- You would better understand the difference between enhancement and change—the former meaning that something becomes *better* than before, the latter simply that it becomes *different*.
- You would be better informed about products and procedures that claim to contribute to your enhanced appearance and health.
- You would be introduced to the time-tested ideas and ideals that my colleagues and I have learned from our mentors, from the annals of historical medical science, and from the more than four decades I have spent caring for more than twenty thousand patients since I became a proud member of the appearance- and health-enhancement profession.

- You would come away with insights that might not have been provided to you previously and a new outlook on the mind-set, procedures, and products necessary for you to recognize and develop the talents that lead to success.
- You would gain a broader understanding of the things you can—and must—do to discover the talents you were given at the time of your birth.
- You would advance mentally, physically, and spiritually in a world brimming with opportunity—but only for those of us who know how to identify, pursue, embrace, and multiply the available resources.
- You would better understand how to convert imaginative thoughts into productive action.
- You would learn how to develop a comprehensive life plan based on the talents you identify in yourself and your realistic limitations, which you must also identify and accept.
- You would know how to give yourself the most precious gifts that the spiritual component of any individual should covet each time our spirits pass through this earthly realm of existence.
- You would come to understand that those gifts include—but are not necessarily limited to—health, happiness, industrious longevity, unselfish prosperity, and the peace of mind that you did all you were expected to do in realms not yet understood by even the wisest of our species.
- You would come to recognize the importance of knowledge, wisdom, and grit in seeing your life plan come to fruition.
- You would become an expert in self-mastery—the ability to take control of your thoughts and actions.
- You would come to understand how your "body is the servant of your mind."[14]

---

14. James Allen, *As a Man Thinketh* (1902; Adelaide, South Australia: University of Adelaide Library, 2015), https://ebooks.adelaide.edu.au/a/allen/james/as-a-man-thinketh/.

- You would recognize the relevance of dwelling on positive, healthy thoughts that direct your body, mind, and spirit toward becoming the best that each is capable of becoming.
- You would be inclined to embrace the mind-set I advise in order to become the most attractive, most perceptive, most focused, most driven, most extraordinary version of yourself possible.
- You would see your self-worth soar to heights never before imagined.
- You would come to like the enhanced image staring back from your mirrors and photographs.
- You would come to realize that you are an integral part of a grand plan in which each of us is expected to excel in all ways possible, as expressed in Luke 12:48.
- You would view the world and the universe around you as an integral part of divinely engineered evolution rather than a hapless victim of consequence or predestination.
- With this renewed sense of *self-worth*, you would feel that *you* are in control of your destiny and the master of yourself.
- As a result, you would be compelled to do whatever you can do to leave the world a better place than it was when the spiritual part of you passed through it this time.

To what greater legacy, what better cause, what better end should any of us commit the talents that were divinely awarded to us?

The gifts (or talents) I have referred to throughout this book are ones that you may or may not choose to accept and multiply. However, if recognized and developed to their maximum potential, they will assist you in overcoming whatever obstacles you encounter on your way to finding your place in the universe.

Once you make the critical choice to develop and diligently follow a personalized life plan that incorporates each of the components I have shared throughout this book, you will have taken the first critical step toward converting positive, preparatory, productive, and prosperous thoughts into actions—actions that produce the kind of results your enlightened mind is now capable of imagining.

The gift that you can give yourself is known by many descriptive terms. For the purposes of this book, I refer to it as "self-care," defined as "the collective ability to choose the thoughts you harbor in your mind and then to convert them into productive actions that benefit your mind, body, and spirit."

The venerable Helen Keller, whom you might recall was left blind and deaf from a childhood illness, often repeated her version of a quotation originally attributed to Edward Everett Hale, an American author and Unitarian clergyman. Helen's version went as follows: "I am only one; but I am one. I cannot do everything; but I can do some things. What I can do, I should do; and with the help of Almighty God, I will do what I can do."

With the assistance of a devoted and skilled mentor, Helen did what she could do. She recognized the remaining talents she possessed, developed them to their maximum potential, and became a highly sought motivational speaker and author on the world stage. I trust that the insights shared throughout this book will encourage you, too, to embrace my recommendations and follow this inspiring mantra. Pledge the following to yourself:

- I am committed to giving myself and the world in which I live the best that I have to offer—as much or as little as it may be.
- I will choose to do the things necessary to enhance my appearance, improve my health, sharpen my mind, and see a bit farther over the horizon so that I might choose only the pathways that will take me to my rightful place in the universe.
- I am now on my way to creating a happier, more productive, and more prosperous life, not only for myself but for those I care about and those who care for me.
- I am committed to doing whatever I can to satisfy the divine directive described in Luke 12:48—"Unto whomsoever much is given, of him shall be much required" (KVJ)—as my spirit is once again tested.

As I have stressed throughout this book, in addition to being able to personally perform many of the appearance-enhancement procedures that might assist you in accomplishing your life plan, I consider my role in that quest to include being your harbinger, your coach, your cheerleader, and your biggest fan. With all those roles in mind, I say this to you. Dream great dreams. Live life to its fullest. Take calculated risks. Surround yourself with trustworthy friends and associates. Never underestimate the power that lies within a resolute mind. Settle for no less than the best you are realistically capable of achieving. And when you have become the person of your dreams, celebrate in the manner that my coach and friend Paul W. "Bear" Bryant advised us players. Do all your celebrating in private, with the people that matter most to you, but when you go out into the world, conduct yourself in the same manner that you would had you not left that arena of competition victorious. Show your class. Never let your highs get too high or your lows too low.

I have also learned that balance and moderation are the keys to everything and that paying forward the gifts given to you should be viewed as both an expectation and a blessing. When good things happen to you, give back. In all ways possible, be a contributor to the human condition so that others might one day stand on your shoulders and peer a bit farther over the horizons that lie before them.

Will you pay what you now know forward, in all the ways you now know how?

That you are reading these final words is a good indication that you will.

As it says on the reverse of the Great Seal of the United States: *Annuit coeptis!* May God continue to favor our undertakings.

Acknowledgments

First and foremost, I wish to acknowledge my wife, Susan N. McCollough, for all her support and encouragement. I want to thank my assistants, Jennifer Arnold and Emily Edmonds. Finally, I extend my thanks to the entire staff and management team at Brown Books and the Agency at Brown Books.

Suggested Reading

Andrews, Andy. *The Bottom of the Pool.* Nashville: W Publishing Group, 2019.

———. *The Noticer: Sometimes, All a Person Needs Is a Little Perspective.* Nashville: Thomas Nelson, 2009.

Buffington, Perry W. *Your Behavior Is Showing: Forty Prescriptions for Understanding and Liking Yourself.* Nashville: Hillbrook House, 1988.

Duckworth, Angela. *Grit: The Power of Passion and Perseverance.* New York: Scribner, 2016.

McCollough, E. Gaylon. *The Appearance Factor.* Gulf Shores, AL: Compass Press, 2016.

———. *Let Us Make Man.* Gulf Shores, AL: Compass Press, 2007.

———. *The Elite Facial Plastic Surgery Practice: Development and Management.* New York: Thieme Medical Publishers, 2017.

———. "The McCollough Condition-Specific Facial Rejuvenation System." *Facial Plastic Surgery* 27 (2011): 112–123.

———. *Victory in the Game of Life: A Paul W. Bryant Alumni-Athlete's Journey.* Gulf Shores, AL: Compass Press, 2018.

About the Author

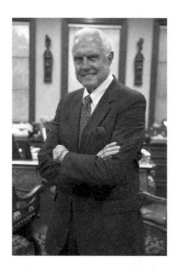

E. Gaylon McCollough, MD, FACS, is an internationally recognized and board-certified surgeon and teacher. The founder of the American College of Rejuvenology and the McCollough Institute for Appearance and Health, Dr. McCollough has been recognized as one of the preeminent doctors in America. The coauthor of three major textbooks on facial and nasal plastic surgery, over the course of his career, Dr. McCollough has served as president of the American Association of Cosmetic Surgeons and the American Board of Facial Plastic and Reconstructive Surgery and has traveled worldwide, conducting educational seminars for plastic surgeons internationally.

Dr. McCollough is an avid supporter of the University of Alabama, his alma mater and home away from home. Dr. McCollough is actively involved in preparing tomorrow's physicians for the road ahead and making health information more accessible to people from all walks of life.

Dr. McCollough and his wife, Susan, live in Gulf Shores, Alabama. They have two grown children and four grandchildren.